PN Mental Health Nursing
Review Module Edition 9.0

P9-CSA-445

CONTRIBUTORS

Sheryl Sommer, PhD, RN, CNE
VP Nursing Education & Strategy

Janean Johnson, MSN, RN
Nursing Education Strategist

Sherry L. Roper, PhD, RN
Nursing Education Strategist

Karin Roberts, PhD, MSN, RN, CNE
Nursing Education Coordinator

Mendy G. McMichael, DNP, RN
Nursing Education Specialist and Content Project Coordinator

Marsha S. Barlow, MSN, RN
Nursing Education Specialist

Norma Jean Henry, MSN/Ed, RN
Nursing Education Specialist

EDITORIAL AND PUBLISHING

Derek Prater
Spring Lenox
Michelle Renner
Mandy Tallmadge
Kelly Von Lunen

CONSULTANTS

Deb Johnson-Schuh, RN, MSN, CNE
Loraine White, RN, BSN, MA

Intellectual Property Notice

Important Notice to the Reader

User's Guide

Welcome to the Assessment Technologies Institute® PN Mental Health Review Module Edition 9.0. The mission of ATI's Content Mastery Series® review modules is to provide user-friendly compendiums of nursing knowledge that will:

- Help you locate important information quickly.

- Assist in your learning efforts.

- Provide exercises for applying your nursing knowledge.

- Facilitate your entry into the nursing profession as a newly licensed PN.

Organization

This review module is organized into units covering foundations for mental health nursing, traditional nonpharmacological therapies, psychobiologic disorders, psychopharmacological therapies, special populations, and psychiatric emergencies. Chapters within these units conform to one of four organizing principles for presenting the content:

- Nursing concepts

- Procedures

- Disorders

- Medications

Nursing concepts chapters begin with an overview describing the central concept and its relevance to nursing. Subordinate themes are covered in outline form to demonstrate relationships and present the information in a clear, succinct manner.

Procedures chapters include an overview describing the procedure(s) covered in the chapter. These chapters will provide you with nursing knowledge relevant to each procedure, including indications, interpretations of findings, nursing actions, and complications.

Disorders chapters include an overview describing the disorder. These chapters cover data collection, including risk factors, subjective data, and objective data, and patient-centered care, including nursing care, medications, teamwork and collaboration, and therapeutic procedures.

Medications chapters include an overview describing a disorder or group of disorders. Medications used to treat these disorders are grouped according to classification. A specific medication may be selected as a prototype or example of the characteristics of medications in this classification. These sections include information about how the medication works, its therapeutic uses, and routes of administration. Next, you will find information about complications, contraindications, and medication and food interactions, as well as nursing interventions and client education to help prevent and/or manage these issues. Finally, the chapter includes information on nursing administration of the medication and evaluation of the medication's effectiveness.

Application Exercises

Questions are provided at the end of each chapter so you can practice applying your knowledge. The Application Exercises include NCLEX-style questions, such as multiple-choice and multiple-select items, and questions that ask you to apply your knowledge in other formats, such as by using an ATI Active Learning Template. After the Application Exercises, an answer key is provided, along with rationales for the answers.

NCLEX® Connections

To prepare for the NCLEX-PN, it is important for you to understand how the content in this review module is connected to the NCLEX-PN test plan. You can find information on the detailed test plan at the National Council of State Boards of Nursing's Web site: https://www.ncsbn.org/. When reviewing content in this review module, regularly ask yourself, "How does this content fit into the test plan, and what types of questions related to this content should I expect?"

To help you in this process, we've included NCLEX Connections at the beginning of each unit and with each question in the Application Exercises Answer Keys. The NCLEX Connections at the beginning of each unit will point out areas of the detailed test plan that relate to the content within the section or unit. The NCLEX Connections attached to the Application Exercises Answer Keys will demonstrate how each exercise fits within the detailed content outline.

These NCLEX Connections will help you understand how the detailed content outline is organized, starting with major client needs categories and subcategories and followed by related content areas and tasks. The major client needs categories are:

- Safe and Effective Care Environment
  - Coordinated Care
  - Safety and Infection Control
- Health Promotion and Maintenance
- Psychosocial Integrity
- Physiological Integrity
  - Basic Care and Comfort
  - Pharmacological Therapies
  - Reduction of Risk Potential
  - Physiological Adaptation

An NCLEX Connection might, for example, alert you that content within a unit is related to:

- Psychosocial Integrity
  - Behavioral Interventions
    - Incorporate behavioral management techniques when caring for a client.

QSEN Competencies

As you use the review modules, you will note the integration of the Quality and Safety Education for Nurses (QSEN) competencies throughout the chapters. These competencies are integral components of the curriculum of many nursing programs in the United States and prepare you to provide safe, high-quality care as a newly licensed PN. Icons appear to draw your attention to the six QSEN competencies:

- Safety: The minimization of risk factors that could cause injury or harm while promoting quality care and maintaining a secure environment for clients, self, and others.
- Patient-Centered Care: The provision of caring and compassionate, culturally sensitive care that addresses clients' physiological, psychological, sociological, spiritual, and cultural needs, preferences, and values.
- Evidence-Based Practice: The use of current knowledge from research and other credible sources, on which to base clinical judgment and client care.
- Informatics: The use of information technology as a communication and information-gathering tool that supports clinical decision-making and scientifically based nursing practice.
- Quality Improvement: Care related and organizational processes that involve the development and implementation of a plan to improve health care services and better meet clients' needs.
- Teamwork and Collaboration: The delivery of client care in partnership with multidisciplinary members of the health care team to achieve continuity of care and positive client outcomes.

Icons

Icons are used throughout the review module to draw your attention to particular areas. Keep an eye out for these icons:

 This icon is used for NCLEX connections.

 This icon is used for content related to safety and is a QSEN competency. When you see this icon, take note of safety concerns or steps that nurses can take to ensure client safety and a safe environment.

 This icon is a QSEN competency that indicates the importance of a holistic approach to providing care.

 This icon, a QSEN competency, points out the integration of research into clinical practice.

 This icon is a QSEN competency and highlights the use of information technology to support nursing practice.

 This icon is used to focus on the QSEN competency of integrating planning processes to meet clients' needs.

 This icon highlights the QSEN competency of care delivery using an interprofessional approach.

 This icon indicates that a media supplement, such as a graphic, animation, or video, is available. If you have an electronic copy of the review module, this icon will appear alongside clickable links to media supplements. If you have a hardcopy version of the review module, visit www.atitesting.com for details on how to access these features.

Feedback

ATI welcomes feedback regarding this review module. Please provide comments to: comments@atitesting.com.

TABLE OF CONTENTS

UNIT 1   Foundations for Mental Health Nursing

CHAPTERS
› Basic Mental Health Nursing Concepts
› Legal and Ethical Issues
› Effective Communication
› Stress and Defense Mechanisms
› Creating and Maintaining a Therapeutic and Safe Environment
› Diverse Practice Settings

NCLEX® CONNECTIONS

When reviewing the chapters in this unit, keep in mind the relevant sections of the NCLEX® outline, in particular:

Client Needs: Coordinated Care

› Relevant topics/tasks include:
  » Advocacy
    › Advocate for the client's rights or needs.
  » Client Rights
    › Recognize the client's right to refuse treatment or procedures.
  » Collaboration with Interdisciplinary Team
    › Identify the need for a nursing or interdisciplinary client care conference.
  » Confidentiality/Information Security
    › Maintain the client's confidentiality.
  » Ethical Practice
    › Intervene to promote ethical practice.
  » Legal Responsibilities
    › Identify legal issues affecting the staff and the client.

Client Needs: Safety and Infection Control

› Relevant topics/tasks include:
  » Accident/Error/Injury Prevention
    › Monitor the client care environment for safety hazards and report problems to appropriate personnel.
  » Least Restrictive Restraints and Safety Devices
    › Check for proper functioning of restraints and safety devices.

chapter 1

Overview

- Provision of care to clients in mental health settings is based on standards of care set by the American Nurses Association, the American Psychiatric Nurses Association, and the International Society of Psychiatric-Mental Health Nurses. Foundational to this care is the use of the nursing process.
- Nurses working in mental health settings should use the nursing process, as well as a holistic approach (biological, social, psychological, and spiritual aspects) to care for clients.
- Nurses should use various methods to collect data from clients. These methods include observation, interviewing, physical examination, and collaboration.

Data Collection

- Data collection is ongoing and involves monitoring the status of the client with each encounter.
- Psychosocial History
  - Perception of own health, beliefs about illness and wellness
  - Activity/leisure activities, how the client passes time
  - Use of substances/substance use disorder
  - Stress level and coping abilities – usual coping strategies, support systems
  - Cultural beliefs and practices
  - Spiritual beliefs
- Mental Status Examination (MSE)

> **M** View Video: Mental Status Examination

  - Level of consciousness is described using the following terms, and observed behavior included in documentation.
    - Alert – The client is responsive and able to fully respond by opening her eyes and attending to a normal tone of voice and speech. The client answers questions spontaneously and appropriately.
    - Lethargy – The client is able to open her eyes and respond but is drowsy and falls asleep readily.
    - Stupor – The client requires vigorous or painful stimuli (pinching a tendon or rubbing the sternum) to elicit a brief response. She may not be able to respond verbally.
    - Coma – No response can be achieved from repeated painful stimuli.
      - Abnormal posturing in the client who is comatose
        - Decorticate rigidity – flexion and internal rotation of upper-extremity joints and legs
        - Decerebrate rigidity – neck and elbow extension, wrist and finger flexion

- ○ Physical appearance
  - ▪ Examination includes observation of personal hygiene, grooming, and clothing choice. Expected findings are that the client is well-kept, clean, and dressed appropriately for the given environment.
- ○ Behavior
  - ▪ Examination includes observation of voluntary and involuntary body movements, and eye contact.
    - ▫ Mood – A client's mood provides information about the emotion that she is feeling.
    - ▫ Affect – A client's affect is an objective expression of mood, such as a flat affect or a lack of facial expression.
- ○ Cognitive and intellectual abilities
  - ▪ Collect data regarding the client's orientation to time, person, and place.
  - ▪ Check the client's memory, both recent and remote.
    - ▫ Immediate – Ask the client to repeat a series of numbers or a list of objects.
    - ▫ Recent – Ask the client to recall recent events, such as visitors from the current day, or the purpose of the current mental health appointment or admission.
    - ▫ Remote – Ask the client to state a fact from his past that is verifiable, such as his birth date or his mother's maiden name.
  - ▪ Check the client's level of knowledge. For example, ask him what he knows about his current illness or hospitalization.
  - ▪ Collect data regarding the client's ability to calculate. For example, can he count backward from 100 in serials of 7?
  - ▪ Check the client's ability to think abstractly. For example, can he interpret a cliché such as, "A bird in the hand is worth two in the bush"? The ability to interpret this demonstrates a higher-level thought process.
  - ▪ Perform an objective data collection regarding of the client's perception of his illness.
  - ▪ Check the client's judgment based on his answer to a hypothetical question. For example, how would he answer the question, "What would you do if there were a fire in your room?" His response to the question should be logical.
  - ▪ Collect data about the client's rate and volume of speech, as well as the quality of his language. His speech should be articulate and his responses meaningful and appropriate.
- • Standardized Screening Tools

  - ○ Mini-Mental State Examination
    - ▪ This examination is used to objectively collect data about a client's cognitive status by evaluating the following.
      - ▫ Orientation to time and place
      - ▫ Attention span and ability to calculate by counting backward by seven
      - ▫ Registration and recalling of objects
      - ▫ Language, including naming of objects, following of commands, and ability to write
  - ○ Glasgow Coma Scale
    - ▪ This examination is used to obtain baseline data of a client's level of consciousness, and for ongoing monitoring. Eye, verbal, and motor response is evaluated, and a number value based on that response is assigned. The highest value possible is 15, which indicates that the client is awake and responding appropriately. A score of 7 or less indicates that the client is in a coma.

Considerations Across the Lifespan

- Children and Adolescents
  - ○ Data collection includes temperament, social and environmental factors, cultural and religious concerns, and developmental level.
  - ○ Mentally healthy children and adolescents should trust others, view the world as safe, accurately interpret their environments, master developmental tasks, and use appropriate coping skills.
  - ○ Children and adolescents experience some of the same mental health problems as adults.
  - ○ Mental health and developmental disorders are not always easily diagnosed, potentially resulting in delayed or inadequate treatment interventions. Factors contributing to this include the following.
    - ▪ Lack of the ability or necessary skills to describe what is happening
    - ▪ A wide variation of "normal" behavior, especially in different developmental stages
  - ○ Check this age group for mood; anxiety; developmental, behavioral, and eating disorders; and risk for self-injury or suicide.
  - ○ Use the standardized screening tool, Home, Education/employment, peer group Activities, Drugs, Sexuality, and Suicide/depression (HEADSS) psychosocial assessment, to identify risk factors in the adolescent.
- Older Adults
  - ○ In addition to the previously mentioned examinations, comprehensive data collection of the older adult client includes the following.
    - ▪ Functional ability, such as the ability to get up out of a chair
    - ▪ Economic and social status
    - ▪ Environmental factors, such as stairways in the home, that can affect the client's well-being and lifestyle
    - ▪ Physical examination
  - ○ Standardized screening tools that are appropriate for the older adult population include the following.

    - ▪ Geriatric Depression Scale (short form)
    - ▪ Michigan Alcoholism Screening Test – Geriatric Version
    - ▪ Mini-Mental State Exam
    - ▪ Pain assessments including visual analogue scales, Wong-Baker FACES Pain Rating Scale, the McGill Pain Questionnaire (MPQ), and the Pain Assessment in Advanced Dementia (PAINAD) scale
  - ○ Collect data from all clients, including older adult clients in the following manner.
    - ▪ Use a private, quiet space with adequate lighting to accommodate for impaired vision and hearing.
    - ▪ Make an introduction, and determine the client's name preference.
    - ▪ Stand or sit at the client's level to conduct the interview, rather than standing over a client who is lying in bed or sitting in a chair.

- Use touch to communicate caring as appropriate. However, respect the client's personal space if he does not wish to be touched.
- Be sure to include questions relating to difficulty sleeping, incontinence, falls or other injuries, depression, dizziness, and loss of energy.
- Include the family and significant others as appropriate.
- Obtain a detailed medication history.
- Following the interview, summarize and ask for feedback from the client.

Mental Health Diagnoses

- The *Diagnostic and Statistical Manual of Mental Disorders*, 5th Edition (DSM-5), published by the American Psychiatric Association, is used as a diagnostic tool to identify mental health diagnoses. It is used by mental health professionals for clients who have mental health disorders.

- Nurses use the DSM-5 in the mental health setting to identify diagnoses and diagnostic criteria to guide data collection; to assist with the identification of nursing diagnoses; to assist with the planning of care; and to implement and evaluate care.

Therapeutic Strategies in the Mental Health Setting

MENTAL HEALTH NURSING INTERVENTIONS	
Counseling	› Using therapeutic communication skills › Assisting with problem solving › Crisis intervention › Stress management
Milieu therapy	› Orienting the client to the physical setting › Identifying rules and boundaries of the setting › Ensuring a safe environment for the client › Assisting the client to participate in appropriate activities
Promotion of self-care activities	› Offering assistance with self-care tasks › Allowing time for the client to complete self-care tasks › Setting incentives to promote client self-care
Psychobiological interventions	› Administering prescribed medications › Reinforcing teaching to the client/family about medications › Monitoring for adverse effects and effectiveness of pharmacological therapy
Cognitive and behavioral therapies	› Modeling › Operant conditioning › Systematic desensitization
Health teaching	› Encouraging social and coping skills
Health promotion and health maintenance	› Assisting the client with cessation of smoking › Monitoring other health conditions
Case management	› Coordinating holistic care to include medical, mental health, and social services

APPLICATION EXERCISES

1. A nurse is discussing mental status examinations with a newly licensed nurse. Which of the following statements by the newly licensed nurse indicates a need for further teaching?

    A. "To check cognitive ability, I should ask the client to count backward by 7."

    B. "To check affect, I should observe the client's facial expression."

    C. "To check language ability, I should instruct the client to write a sentence."

    D. "To check remote memory, I should have the client repeat a list of objects."

2. A nurse is assisting in the planning of care for a client who has a mental health disorder. Which of the following is appropriate to include as a psychobiological intervention?

    A. Assist the client with systematic desensitization therapy.

    B. Encourage the client to use appropriate coping mechanisms.

    C. Evaluate the client for comorbid health conditions.

    D. Monitor the client for adverse effects of medications.

3. A nurse in an outpatient mental health clinic is preparing to conduct an initial client interview. When conducting the interview, which of the following is the highest priority action?

    A. Respect the client's need for personal space.

    B. Identify the client's perception of her mental health status.

    C. Include the client's family in the interview.

    D. Reinforce teaching about the client's mental health disorder.

4. A nurse is told during change-of-shift report that a client is stuporous. When collecting data from the client, which of the following is an expected finding?

    A. The client arouses briefly in response to a sternal rub.

    B. The client has a Glasgow Coma Scale score less than 7.

    C. The client exhibits decorticate rigidity.

    D. The client is alert but disoriented to time and place.

5. A nurse is assisting with the planning of a peer group discussion about the *Diagnostic and Statistical Manual of Mental Disorders*, 5th Edition (DSM-5). Which of the following is appropriate to include in the discussion? (Select all that apply.)

_____ A. The DSM-5 is used to identify mental health disorders.

_____ B. The DSM-5 establishes diagnostic criteria.

_____ C. The DSM-5 indicates recommended pharmacological treatment.

_____ D. The DSM-5 is used to assist in the planning of care.

_____ E. The DSM-5 indicates expected data collection findings.

6. A charge nurse is discussing therapeutic strategies in the mental health setting with a newly licensed nurse. Use the ATI Active Learning Template: Basic Concept to complete this item to identify at least three specific nursing interventions for counseling and milieu therapy.

APPLICATION EXERCISES KEY

1. A. INCORRECT: This statement does not require further teaching. Counting backward by 7 is an appropriate technique to check a client's cognitive ability.

    B. INCORRECT: This statement does not require further teaching. Observing a client's facial expression is appropriate when checking affect.

    C. INCORRECT: This statement does not require further teaching. Writing a sentence is an indication of language ability.

    D. **CORRECT:** This statement requires further teaching. Asking the client to repeat a list of objects is appropriate to check immediate, rather than remote, memory.

    🅝 NCLEX® Connection: Psychosocial Integrity, Mental Health Concepts

2. A. INCORRECT: Assisting with systematic desensitization therapy is a cognitive and behavioral, rather than psychobiological, intervention.

    B. INCORRECT: Encouraging appropriate coping mechanisms is a counseling or health teaching, rather than a psychobiological intervention.

    C. INCORRECT: Evaluating for comorbid health conditions is health promotion and maintenance, rather than a psychobiological intervention.

    D. **CORRECT:** Monitoring for adverse effects of medications is an example of a psychobiological intervention.

    🅝 NCLEX® Connection: Psychosocial Integrity, Mental Health Concepts

3. A. INCORRECT: It is appropriate to respect the client's need for personal space. However, it is not the highest priority action when taking the nursing process approach to client care.

    B. **CORRECT:** Data collection is the priority action when taking the nursing process approach to client care. Identifying the client's perception of her mental health status provides important information about the client's psychosocial history.

    C. INCORRECT: If the client wishes, it is appropriate to include the client's family in the interview. However, it is not the highest priority action when taking the nursing process approach to client care.

    D. INCORRECT: It is appropriate to reinforce teaching for the client about her disorder. However, it is not the highest priority action when taking the nursing process approach to client care.

    🅝 NCLEX® Connection: Psychosocial Integrity, Mental Health Concepts

4. A. **CORRECT:** A client who is stuporous requires vigorous or painful stimuli to elicit a response.

    B. INCORRECT: A GCS score of less than 7 indicates a comatose, rather than stuporous, level of consciousness.

    C. INCORRECT: Abnormal posturing is associated with a comatose, rather than stuporous, level of consciousness.

    D. INCORRECT: A client who is stuporous is not alert.

    Ⓝ NCLEX® Connection: Psychosocial Integrity, Mental Health Concepts

5. A. **CORRECT:** The DSM-5 is used as a diagnostic tool to identify mental health diagnoses.

    B. **CORRECT:** The DSM-5 establishes diagnostic criteria for mental health disorders.

    C. INCORRECT: The DSM-5 is a diagnostic tool for the diagnosis of mental health disorders but does not indicate pharmacological treatment.

    D. **CORRECT:** Nurses use the DSM-5 to assist in the planning of care, and to implement and evaluate care.

    E. **CORRECT:** The DSM-5 identifies expected findings for mental health disorders.

    Ⓝ NCLEX® Connection: Psychosocial Integrity, Mental Health Concepts

6. *Using ATI Active Learning Template: Basic Concept*
    - Nursing Interventions
      - Counseling
        - Using therapeutic communication skills
        - Assisting with problem solving
        - Crisis intervention
        - Stress management
      - Milieu Therapy
        - Orienting the client to the physical setting
        - Identifying rules and boundaries of the setting
        - Ensuring a safe environment for the client
        - Assisting the client to participate in appropriate activities

    Ⓝ NCLEX® Connection: Psychosocial Integrity, Therapeutic Environment

chapter 2

Overview

- A nurse who works in the mental health setting is responsible for practicing ethically, competently, safely, and in a manner consistent with all local, state, and federal laws.
- Nurses must have an understanding of ethical principles and how they apply when providing care for clients in mental health settings.
- Nurses are responsible for understanding and protecting client rights.

Legal Rights of Clients in the Mental Health Setting

- Clients who have been diagnosed and/or hospitalized with a mental health disorder are guaranteed the same civil rights as any other citizen.
  - The right to humane treatment and care, such as medical and dental care
  - The right to vote
  - The right to due process of law, including the right to press legal charges against another person
- Clients also have various specific rights.
  - Informed consent and the right to refuse treatment
  - Confidentiality
  - A written plan of care/treatment that includes discharge follow-up, as well as participation in the care plan and review of that plan
  - Communication with people outside the mental health facility, including family members, attorneys, and other health care professionals
  - Provision of adequate interpretive services if needed
  - Care provided with respect, dignity, and without discrimination
  - Freedom from harm related to physical or pharmacologic restraint, seclusion, and any physical or mental abuse or neglect
  - Provision of care with the least restrictive interventions necessary to meet the client's needs without allowing him to be a threat to himself or others
- Some legal issues regarding health care can be decided in court using a specialized civil category called a tort. A tort is a wrongful act or injury committed by an entity or person against another person or another person's property. Torts can be used to decide liability issues, as well as intentional issues that can involve criminal penalties, such as abuse of a client.
- State laws can vary greatly. The nurse must be aware of specific laws regarding client care within the state or states in which the nurse practices.

Ethical Issues for Clients in the Mental Health Setting

- In comparison to laws, statutes, and regulations (enacted by local, state, or federal government), ethical issues are philosophical ideas regarding right and wrong.
- Nurses are frequently confronted with ethical dilemmas regarding client care (bioethical issues).
- Because ethics are philosophical and involve values and morals, there is frequently no clear-cut, simple resolution to an ethical dilemma.
- Ethical principles must be used to decide ethical issues.

ETHICAL PRINCIPLE	DEFINITION	EXAMPLE
Beneficence	› This relates to the quality of doing good and can be described as charity.	› A nurse helps a newly admitted client who has psychosis feel safe in the environment of the mental health facility.
Autonomy	› This refers to the client's right to make her own decisions. But the client must accept the consequences of those decisions. The client also must respect the decisions of others.	› Rather than giving advice to a client who has difficulty making decisions, a nurse helps the client explore all alternatives and arrive at a choice.
Justice	› This is fair and equal treatment for all.	› During a treatment team meeting, a nurse collaborates with the interdisciplinary team regarding whether or not two clients who broke the same facility rule were treated equally.
Fidelity	› This relates to loyalty and faithfulness to the client and to one's duty.	› A client asks a nurse to be present when he talks to his mother for the first time in a year. The nurse remains with the client during this interaction.
Veracity	› This refers to being honest when dealing with a client.	› A client states, "You and that other staff member were talking about me, weren't you?" The nurse truthfully replies, "We were discussing ways to help you relate to the other clients in a more positive way."

Confidentiality

- The client's right to privacy is protected by the Health Insurance Portability and Accountability Act (HIPAA) of 2003.
- It is important to gain an understanding of the federal law and of various state laws as they relate to confidentiality in specific health care facilities.
- Information about the client, verbal and in writing, must be shared only with those who are responsible for implementing the client's treatment plan.
- Information can be shared with other persons not involved in the client treatment plan by client consent only.
- Specific mental health issues include disclosing HIV status, the duty to warn and protect third parties, and the reporting of child and elder abuse.

Resources for Solving Ethical Client Issues

- Code of Ethics for Nurses, found at http://nursingworld.org
- Patient Care Partnership, found at www.aha.org
- Nurse practice act of a specific state
- Legal advice from attorneys
- Facility policies
- Other members of the health care team, including facility bioethics committee (if available)
- Members of the clergy and other spiritual or ethical counselors

Types of Commitment to a Mental Health Facility

- Voluntary commitment – The client or client's guardian chooses commitment to a mental health facility in order to obtain treatment. A voluntarily committed client has the right to apply for release at any time. This client is considered competent, and so has the right to refuse medication and treatment.
- Involuntary (civil) commitment – The client enters the mental health facility against her will for an indefinite period of time. The commitment is based on the client's need for psychiatric treatment, the risk of harm to self or others, or the inability to provide self-care. The need for commitment could be determined by a judge of the court or by another agency. The number of physicians, which is usually two, required to certify that the client's condition requires commitment varies from state to state.

    - Emergency involuntary commitment – A type of involuntary commitment in which the client is hospitalized to prevent harm to self or others. Emergency commitment is usually temporary (up to 10 days). This type of commitment usually is imposed by primary care providers, mental health providers, or police officers.

    - Observational or temporary involuntary commitment – A type of involuntary commitment in which the client is in need of observation, a diagnosis, and a treatment plan. The time for this type of commitment is controlled by state statute and varies greatly between states. This can be imposed by a family member, legal guardian, primary care provider, or a mental health provider.

    - Long-term or formal involuntary commitment – A type of commitment that is similar to temporary commitment but must be imposed by the courts. Time of commitment varies, but is usually 60 to 180 days. Sometimes, there is no set release date.

    - Clients admitted under involuntary commitment are still considered competent and have the right to refuse treatment, unless they have gone through a legal competency hearing and have been judged incompetent. The client who has been judged incompetent has a temporary or permanent guardian, usually a family member if possible, appointed by the court. The guardian can sign informed consent for the client. The guardian is expected to consider what the client would want if he were still competent.

Client Rights Regarding Seclusion and Restraint

- Nurses must follow federal/state/facility policies that govern the use of restraints.
- Use of seclusion rooms and/or restraints can be warranted and authorized for clients in some cases.
- In general, seclusion and/or restraint should be ordered for the shortest duration necessary, and only if less restrictive measures are not sufficient. They are for the physical protection of the client, other clients, and/or staff.
- A client can request voluntary temporary seclusion in cases in which the environment is disturbing or seems too stimulating.
- Restraints can be either physical or chemical, such as neuroleptic medication to calm the client.
- Seclusion and/or restraint must never be used for:
  - Convenience of the staff.
  - Punishment of the client.
  - Clients who are extremely physically or mentally unstable.
  - Clients who cannot tolerate the decreased stimulation of a seclusion room.
- When all other less restrictive means have been tried to prevent a client from harming self or others, the following must occur in order for seclusion or restraint to be used.
  - The treatment must be ordered by the primary care provider in writing.
  - The order must specify the duration of treatment.
  - The provider must rewrite the order, specifying the type of restraint, every 24 hr or the frequency of time specified by facility policy.

  - Nursing responsibilities must be identified in the protocol, including how often the client should be:
    - Monitored (including for safety and physical needs), and the client's behavior documented.
    - Offered food and fluid.
    - Toileted.
    - Monitored for vital signs.
  - Complete documentation includes a description of the following.
    - Precipitating events and behavior of the client prior to seclusion or restraint
    - Alternative actions taken to avoid seclusion or restraint
    - The time treatment began
    - The client's current behavior, what foods or fluids were offered and taken, needs provided for, and vital signs
    - Medication administration
- An emergency situation must be present for the nurse to use seclusion or restraints without first obtaining a provider's written order. If this treatment is initiated, the nurse must obtain the written order within a specified period of time (usually 15 to 30 min).

Tort Law in the Mental Health Setting

- Although intentional torts can occur in any health care setting, they are particularly likely to occur in mental health settings due to the increased likelihood of violence and client behavior that can be challenging to facility staff.

INTENTIONAL TORT	EXAMPLE
False imprisonment	› Confining a client to a specific area, such as a seclusion room, is false imprisonment if the reason for such confinement is for the convenience of the staff.
Assault	› Making a threat to a client's person, such as approaching the client in a threatening manner with a syringe in hand, is considered assault.
Battery	› Touching a client in a harmful or offensive way is considered battery. This would occur if the nurse threatening the client with a syringe actually grabbed the client and gave an injection.

Documentation

- It is vital to clearly and objectively document information related to violent or other unusual episodes. The nurse should document:
  - ○ Client behavior in a clear and objective manner.
    - ▪ Example: The client suddenly began to run down the hall with both hands in the air, screaming obscenities.
  - ○ Staff response to disruptive, violent, or potentially harmful behavior, such as suicide threats or potential or actual harm to others, including timelines and the extent of response.
    - ▪ Example: The client states, "I'm going to pound (other client) into the ground." Client has picked up a chair and is standing 3 feet from other client with chair held over his head in both hands. Nurse calls for help. Client is immediately told by nurse, "Put down the chair, and back away from (the other person)." Other client moved away to safe area. Five other staff members respond to verbal call for help within 30 seconds and stood several yards from client. Client then put the chair down, quietly turned around, walked to his room, and sat on the bed.

APPLICATION EXERCISES

1. A nurse is discussing candidates for emergency admission to a mental health facility with a newly licensed nurse. Which of the following is an example of a client who requires emergency admission to a mental health facility?

    A. A client who has schizophrenia and has frequent hallucinations

    B. A client who has symptoms of depression and attempted suicide a year ago

    C. A client who has borderline personality disorder and assaulted a homeless man with a metal rod

    D. A client who has bipolar disorder and paces quickly down the sidewalk while talking to himself

2. A client tells a student nurse, "Don't tell anyone, but I hid a sharp knife under my mattress in order to protect myself from my roommate, who is always yelling at me and threatening me." Which of the following actions should the nurse take?

    A. Keep the client's communication confidential, but talk to the client daily, using therapeutic communication to convince him to admit to hiding the knife.

    B. Keep the client's communication confidential, but watch the client and his roommate closely.

    C. Tell the client that this must be reported to health care staff because it concerns the health and safety of the client and others.

    D. Report the incident, but do not inform the client of the intention to do so.

3. A nurse decides to put a client who has psychosis in seclusion overnight because the unit is very short-staffed and the client frequently fights with other clients. This is an example of

    A. beneficence.

    B. a tort.

    C. a facility policy.

    D. justice.

4. A nurse is caring for a client in restraints. Which of the following statements are appropriate documentation? (Select all that apply.)

    _____ A. "Client ate most of his breakfast."

    _____ B. "Client was offered 8 oz of water every hr."

    _____ C. "Client shouted at assistive personnel."

    _____ D. "Client received chlorpromazine 15 mg by mouth at 1000."

    _____ E. "Client acted out after lunch."

5. A nurse hears a newly licensed nurse discussing a client's hallucinations in the hallway with another nurse. Which of the following actions should the nurse take first?

    A. Notify the nurse manager.

    B. Tell the nurse to stop discussing the behavior.

    C. Assist with providing an in-service program about confidentiality.

    D. Complete an incident report.

6. A nurse in a mental health facility is caring for a client who has bipolar disorder. The client becomes violent and begins throwing objects at other clients. After calling for assistance, what actions should the nurse take next? Use the ATI Active Learning Template: Basic Concept to complete this item to describe at least four nursing interventions with rationales.

APPLICATION EXERCISES KEY

1. A. INCORRECT: The presence of hallucinations does not constitute a clear reason for emergency commitment.

    B. INCORRECT: Clinical findings of depression do not constitute a clear reason for emergency commitment.

    C. **CORRECT:** A client who is a current danger to self or others is a candidate for emergency admission.

    D. INCORRECT: A client who is pacing does not constitute a clear reason for emergency commitment.

    Ⓝ NCLEX® Connection: Psychosocial Integrity, Crisis Intervention

2. A. INCORRECT: The information cannot be kept confidential. Daily therapeutic communication is not an appropriate action to correct the client's behavior.

    B. INCORRECT: The information cannot be kept confidential. Observing the client and his roommate is not an appropriate action.

    C. **CORRECT:** This is a serious safety issue that must be reported to the staff. Using the principle of veracity, the student tells this client truthfully what must be done regarding the issue.

    D. INCORRECT: The client should be aware that the information will be reported to the health care staff.

    Ⓝ NCLEX® Connection: Psychosocial Integrity, Crisis Intervention

3. A. INCORRECT: Beneficence is doing good for a client.

    B. **CORRECT:** A civil wrong that violates a client's civil rights is a tort. In this case, it is false imprisonment.

    C. INCORRECT: If this were a facility policy, it would be a violation of federal and state statute, and the nurse could still be held responsible for following it.

    D. INCORRECT: Justice involves the fair and equal treatment of clients.

    Ⓝ NCLEX® Connection: Coordinated Care, Legal Responsibilities

4. A. INCORRECT: The fact that the client ate most of his breakfast is subjective and should not be documented.

    B. **CORRECT:** How much water was offered and how often it was offered is objective data that should be documented when a nurse is caring for a client in restraints.

    C. **CORRECT:** A description of the client's verbal communication is objective data and should be documented.

    D. **CORRECT:** The dosage and time of medication administration is objective data and should be documented when caring for a client in restraints.

    E. INCORRECT: Acting out is subjective data and therefore should not be documented.

    (N) NCLEX® Connection: Safety and Infection Control, Least Restrictive Restraints and Safety Devices

5. A. INCORRECT: The nurse should notify the nurse manager, but this is not the first action the nurse should take.

    B. **CORRECT:** The nurse should tell the newly licensed nurse to stop discussing the client's hallucinations in a public location. This is the priority action.

    C. INCORRECT: The nurse should assist in providing an in-service program about confidentiality, but this is not the first action the nurse should take.

    D. INCORRECT: The nurse should complete an incident report, but this is not the first action the nurse should take.

    (N) NCLEX® Connection: Coordinated Care, Confidentiality/Information Security

6. *Using the ATI Active Learning Template: Basic Concept*
    - Nursing Interventions
        - Tell the client calmly to sit down. Verbal intervention is the least restrictive method when dealing with an aggressive client.
        - Place the client in a monitored seclusion room. It can become necessary to place the client in seclusion if the client persists in the behavior.
        - Administer diazepam (Valium) intramuscularly. It can be necessary for the nurse to administer diazepam to calm the client.
        - Obtain a prescription for mechanical restraints. It can be necessary for the nurse to contact the provider to obtain a prescription for restraints.

    (N) NCLEX® Connection: Psychosocial Integrity, Behavioral Management

UNIT 1   FOUNDATIONS FOR MENTAL HEALTH NURSING

CHAPTER 3   Effective Communication

Overview

- Communication is a complex process of sending, receiving, and comprehending messages between two or more people. It is a dynamic and ongoing process that creates a unique experience between the participants.
  - ○ Communicating effectively is a skill that can be developed.
  - ○ Nurses use communication when providing care to establish relationships, demonstrate caring, obtain information, and assist with changing behaviors.
  - ○ Therapeutic communication is foundational to the nurse-client relationship.

Basic Communication

- Primary Levels of Basic Communication
  - ○ Intrapersonal communication – Occurs within an individual, also identified as "self-talk." This is the internal discussion that takes place when an individual is thinking thoughts and not outwardly verbalizing them. In nursing, intrapersonal communication allows the nurse to collect data from a client or situation and critically think about the client/situation before communicating verbally.
  - ○ Interpersonal communication – Occurs between two or more people in a small group. This is the most common form of communication in nursing and requires an exchange of information with an individual or small group.
  - ○ Public communication – Occurs within large groups of people. In nursing, this commonly occurs during educational endeavors where the nurse is educating a large group of individuals, such as in a community setting.
  - ○ Transpersonal communication – Addresses an individual's spiritual needs and provides interventions to meet those needs.

- Verbal Communication

CONTENT OF THE MESSAGE	IMPACT ON THE COMMUNICATION
› Vocabulary – These are the words that are used to communicate either a written or a spoken message.	› Limited vocabulary or speaking a language other than English can make it difficult for the nurse to communicate with the client. Use of medical jargon can decrease client understanding.
› Denotative/connotative meaning – When communicating, participants must share meanings.	› Words that have multiple meanings can cause miscommunication if they are interpreted differently.
› Clarity/brevity – The shortest, simplest communication is usually most effective.	› Communication that is long and complex can be difficult to understand.
› Timing/relevance – Knowing when to communicate allows the receiver to be more attentive to the message.	› Communicating with a client who is in pain or distracted will make it difficult for the message to be conveyed.
› Pacing – The rate of speech can communicate a meaning to the receiver.	› Speaking rapidly can communicate the impression that the nurse is in a rush and does not have time for the client.
› Intonation – The tone of voice can communicate a variety of feelings.	› The nurse can communicate feelings, such as acceptance, judgment, and dislike through tone of voice.

- Nonverbal Communication
    - Nurses should be aware of how they communicate nonverbally. The nurse should encourage clients' appropriate use of nonverbal communication, remembering that culture affects interpretation. Attention to the following behaviors is important, as it is compared to the verbal message being conveyed.
        - Appearance
        - Posture
        - Gait
        - Facial expressions
        - Eye contact
        - Gestures
        - Sounds
        - Territoriality
        - Personal space
        - Silence

Therapeutic Communication

- Therapeutic communication is the purposeful use of communication to build and maintain helping relationships with clients, families, and significant others.

- The nurse uses interactive, purposeful communication skills to:
  - Elicit and attend to the client's thoughts, feelings, concerns, and needs.
  - Express empathy and genuine concern for the client's and family's issues.
  - Obtain information and give feedback about the client's condition.
  - Intervene to promote functional behavior and effective interpersonal relationships.
  - Monitor and document the client's progress toward goals and outcomes.

- Children and older adults frequently require altered techniques to enhance communication.

- Use of the nursing process depends on therapeutic communication between the nurse, client, client's family, and interprofessional team.

- Characteristics of Therapeutic Communication
  - Client centered – not social or reciprocal
  - Purposeful, planned, and goal-directed

- Essential Components of Therapeutic Communication
  - Time – Plan for and allow adequate time to communicate.
  - Attending behaviors or active listening – These are nonverbal means of conveying interest in another person.
    - Eye contact typically conveys interest and respect, but varies by situation and culture.
    - Body language and posture can demonstrate level of comfort and ease.
    - Vocal quality enhances rapport and emphasizes particular topics or issues.
    - Verbal tracking provides feedback by restating or summarizing a client's statements.
  - Caring attitude – Show concern and facilitate an emotional connection with the client and the client's family.
  - Honesty – Be open, direct, truthful, and sincere.
  - Trust – Demonstrate reliability without doubt or question.
  - Empathy – Convey an objective awareness and understanding of the feelings, emotions, and behaviors of others, including trying to envision what it must be like to be in the position of the client and the client's family.
  - Nonjudgmental attitude – This is a display of acceptance that will encourage open, honest communication.

 View Video: Therapeutic and Nontherapeutic Communication

Nursing Process

- Data Collection
  - ○ Monitor verbal and nonverbal communication needs.
  - ○ Consider the client's developmental level and how communication should be altered during the assessment phase.
    - Children
      - □ Use simple, straightforward language.
      - □ Nurses should be aware of their own nonverbal messages, as children are sensitive to nonverbal communication.
      - □ Enhance communication by being at the child's eye level.
      - □ Incorporate play in interactions.

    - Older Adults
      - □ Recognize that the client can require amplification.
      - □ Minimize distractions, and face the client when speaking.
      - □ Allow plenty of time for the client to respond.
      - □ When impaired communication is noted, ask for input from caregivers or family to determine the extent of the deficits and how best to communicate.
    - Recognize any cultural considerations that can affect communication.
- Planning
  - ○ Minimize distractions.
  - ○ Provide for privacy.
  - ○ Identify mutually agreed-upon client outcomes.
  - ○ Set priorities according to the client's needs.
  - ○ Plan for adequate time for interventions.
- Implementation
  - ○ Establish a trusting nurse-client relationship. The client feels more at ease during the implementation phase when a helping relationship has been established.
  - ○ Provide empathetic responses and explanations to the client by using observations and providing hope, humor, and information.

Effective Skills and Techniques

EFFECTIVE COMMUNICATION	INFLUENCE ON COMMUNICATION
Silence	› Silence allows time for meaningful reflection.
Active listening	› The nurse is able to hear, observe, and understand what the client communicates and to provide feedback.
Open-ended questions	› This technique facilitates spontaneous responses and interactive discussion.
Clarifying techniques	› These are used to determine if the message received was accurate. » Restating – uses the client's exact words. » Reflecting – directs the focus back to the client in order for the client to examine his feelings. » Paraphrasing – restates the client's feelings and thoughts for the client to confirm what has been communicated. » Exploring – allows the nurse to gather more information regarding important topics mentioned by the client.
Offering general leads, broad opening statements	› This encourages the client to determine where the communication can start and to continue talking.
Showing acceptance and recognition	› This technique acknowledges the nurse's interest and nonjudgmental attitude.
Focusing	› Focusing helps the client to concentrate on what is important.
Asking questions	› This is a way to seek additional information.
Giving information	› This provides details that the client can need for decision making.
Presenting reality	› This technique is used to help the client focus on what is actually happening and to dispel delusions, hallucinations, or faulty beliefs.
Summarizing	› Summarizing emphasizes important points and reviews what has been discussed.
Offering self	› This demonstrates a willingness to spend time with the client. Limited personal information can be shared, but the focus should return to the client as soon as possible. Relevant self-disclosure by the nurse allows the client to see that his experience is shared by others and understood.
Touch	› If appropriate, touch communicates caring and can provide comfort to the client.

Barriers to Effective Communication

- Asking irrelevant personal questions
- Offering personal opinions
- Giving advice
- Giving false reassurance
- Minimizing feelings
- Changing the topic
- Asking "why" questions
- Offering value judgments
- Excessive questioning
- Responding approvingly or disapprovingly

APPLICATION EXERCISES

1. A nurse is conducting a class on therapeutic communication to a group of newly licensed nurses. Which of the following responses regarding nonverbal communication by a newly licensed nurse requires additional teaching?

    A. Personal space

    B. Posture

    C. Eye contact

    D. Intonation

2. A nurse is communicating with a client on the acute mental health facility. The client states, "I can't sleep. I stay up all night." The nurse responds, "You are having difficulty sleeping?" Which of the following therapeutic communication techniques is the nurse demonstrating?

    A. Offering general leads

    B. Summarizing

    C. Focusing

    D. Restating

3. A nurse is communicating with a newly admitted client. Which of the following is a barrier to therapeutic communication?

    A. Offering advice

    B. Reflecting meaning

    C. Listening attentively

    D. Giving information

4. A nurse is conducting therapy with a several clients and their families. Effective communication with clients and families is based on

    A. discussing in-depth topics with which the client feels comfortable.

    B. using silence to avoid unpleasant or difficult topics.

    C. attending to verbal and nonverbal behaviors.

    D. requiring the client and family to ask for feedback.

5. When a family asks a nurse for reassurance about a client's condition, which of the following is an appropriate response?

      A. "I think your son is getting better. What have you noticed?"

      B. "I'm sure everything will be okay. It just takes time to heal."

      C. "I'm not sure what's wrong. Have you asked the doctor about your concerns?"

      D. "I understand you're concerned. Let's discuss what concerns you specifically."

6. A nurse in a mental health facility is preparing to conduct a class on grief and loss with older adult clients. Use the ATI Active Learning Template: Basic Concept to complete this item to describe at least four verbal or nonverbal communication needs the nurse should consider when working with older adult clients.

APPLICATION EXERCISES KEY

1. A. INCORRECT: Personal space is a part of nonverbal behavior and should be included in the teaching.

    B. INCORRECT: Posture is a part of nonverbal behavior and should be included in the teaching.

    C. INCORRECT: Eye contact is a part of nonverbal behavior and should be included in the teaching.

    D. **CORRECT:** Intonation is the tone of one's voice and can communicate a variety of feelings.

    Ⓝ NCLEX® Connection: Psychosocial Integrity, Therapeutic Communication

2. A. INCORRECT: Offering general leads allows the nurse to take the direction of the discussion.

    B. INCORRECT: Summarizing enables the nurse to bring together important points of discussion to enhance understanding.

    C. INCORRECT: Focusing concentrates the attention on a single point.

    D. **CORRECT:** Restating allows the nurse to repeat the main idea expressed.

    Ⓝ NCLEX® Connection: Psychosocial Integrity, Therapeutic Communication

3. A. **CORRECT:** Offering advice to a client is a barrier to therapeutic communication and should be avoided. Advice tends to interfere with the client's ability to make personal decisions and choices.

    B. INCORRECT: Reflection encourages the client to make choices and is therapeutic.

    C. INCORRECT: Listening is an important therapeutic technique.

    D. INCORRECT: Giving information informs the client of needed facts.

    Ⓝ NCLEX® Connection: Psychosocial Integrity, Therapeutic Communication

4. A. INCORRECT: In-depth conversations are not necessary for effective communication. Often, very brief conversations are most effective.

    B. INCORRECT: The purpose of effective silence is to allow the client time for reflection or to convey nonverbal support. It is not used to avoid unpleasant or difficult topics.

    C. **CORRECT:** Attending to verbal and nonverbal behaviors is necessary for effective communication.

    D. INCORRECT: Requiring the client and family to ask for feedback is not an effective technique.

    Ⓝ NCLEX® Connection: Psychosocial Integrity, Therapeutic Communication

5. A. INCORRECT: This interjects the nurse's opinion and can cause the family members to withhold their thoughts and feelings.

    B. INCORRECT: This interjects the nurse's opinion and can cause the family members to withhold their thoughts and feelings.

    C. INCORRECT: This interjects the nurse's opinion and can cause the family members to withhold their thoughts and feelings.

    D. **CORRECT:** A therapeutic response reflects upon and accepts the family's feelings, and it allows the members to clarify what they are feeling.

    Ⓝ NCLEX® Connection: Psychosocial Integrity, Therapeutic Communication

6. *Using the ATI Active Learning Template: Basic Concept*
    - Recognize that the client can require amplification.
    - Minimize distractions, and face the client when speaking.
    - Allow plenty of time for the client to respond.
    - When impaired communication is noted, ask for input from caregivers or family to determine the extent of the deficits and how best to communicate.

    Ⓝ NCLEX® Connection: Psychosocial Integrity, Therapeutic Communication

UNIT 1   FOUNDATIONS FOR MENTAL HEALTH NURSING

CHAPTER 4   Stress and Defense Mechanisms

Overview

- Stress can result from a change in one's environment that is threatening, causes challenges, or is perceived as damaging to that person's well-being. Stress causes anxiety.
- Dysfunctional behavior can occur when a defense mechanism is used as a response to anxiety.
- Individuals can use defense mechanisms as a way to manage conflict in response to anxiety. Defense mechanisms are reversible, and can be adaptive or maladaptive.
  - Adaptive use of defense mechanisms helps people to achieve their goals in acceptable ways. Defense mechanisms become maladaptive when they interfere with functioning, relationships, and orientation to reality.
  - It is important that the defense mechanism used is appropriate to the situation, and that an individual uses a variety of defense mechanisms, rather than having the same reaction to every situation.

Defense Mechanisms

- Altruism and sublimation are defense mechanisms that are always healthy. Other defense mechanisms can be used in a healthy manner. However, they can become maladaptive if used inappropriately or repetitively.
- Intermediate defenses include repression, reaction formation, displacement, rationalization, and undoing.
- Immature defenses include projection, dissociation, splitting, and denial.

DEFENSE MECHANISM	DESCRIPTION	EXAMPLE
Altruism	› Dealing with anxiety by reaching out to others	› A nurse who lost a family member in a fire is a volunteer firefighter.
Sublimation	› Dealing with unacceptable feelings or impulses by unconsciously substituting acceptable forms of expression	› A person who has feelings of anger and hostility toward his work supervisor sublimates those feelings by working out vigorously at the gym during his lunch period.
Suppression	› Voluntarily denying unpleasant thoughts and feelings	› A person who has lost his job states he will worry about paying his bills next week.
Repression	› Putting unacceptable ideas, thoughts, and emotions out of conscious awareness	› A person who has a fear of the dentist's drill continually "forgets" his dental appointments.
Displacement	› Shifting feelings related to an object, person, or situation to another less threatening object, person, or situation	› A person who is angry about losing his job destroys his child's favorite toy.

DEFENSE MECHANISM	DESCRIPTION	EXAMPLE
Reaction formation	› Overcompensating or demonstrating the opposite behavior of what is felt	› A person who dislikes her sister's daughter offers to babysit so that her sister can go out of town.
Undoing	› Performing an act to make up for prior behavior	› An adolescent completes his chores without being prompted after having an argument with his parent.
Rationalization	› Creating reasonable and acceptable explanations for unacceptable behavior	› A young adult explains he had to drive home from a party after drinking alcohol because he had to feed his dog.
Dissociation	› Temporarily blocking memories and perceptions from consciousness	› An adolescent witnesses a shooting and is unable to recall any details of the event.
Splitting	› Demonstrating an inability to reconcile negative and positive attributes of self or others	› A client tells a nurse that she is the only one who cares about her, yet the following day, the same client refuses to talk to the nurse.
Projection	› Blaming others for unacceptable thoughts and feelings	› A young adult blames his substance use disorder on his parents' refusal to buy him a new car.
Denial	› Pretending the truth is not reality to manage the anxiety of acknowledging what is real	› A parent who is informed that his son was killed in combat tells everyone he is coming home for the holidays.
Regression	› Demonstrating behavior from an earlier developmental level.Often exhibited as childlike or immature behavior.	› A school-age child begins wetting the bed and sucking his thumb after learning that his parents are separating.

Anxiety

- Anxiety is viewed on a continuum with increasing levels of anxiety leading to decreasing ability to function.

  ○ Normal – A healthy life force that is necessary for survival, normal anxiety motivates people to take action. For example, a potentially violent situation occurs on the mental health unit, and the nurse moves rapidly to defuse the situation. The anxiety experienced by the nurse during the situation helped him perform quickly and efficiently.

  ○ Acute (state) – This level of anxiety is precipitated by an imminent loss or change that threatens one's sense of security. For example, the sudden death of a loved one precipitates an acute state of anxiety.

  ○ Chronic (trait) – This level of anxiety is one that usually develops over time, often starting in childhood. The adult who experiences chronic anxiety can display that anxiety in physical findings, such as fatigue and frequent headaches.

Data Collection

- Observation of a client's level of anxiety is basic to therapeutic intervention in any setting.

LEVELS OF ANXIETY	
Mild	› Mild anxiety occurs in the normal experience of everyday living. › It increases one's ability to perceive reality. › There is an identifiable cause of the anxiety. › Other characteristics include a vague feeling of mild discomfort, restlessness, irritability, impatience, and apprehension. › The client may exhibit behaviors such as finger- or foot-tapping, fidgeting, or lip-chewing as mild tension-relieving behaviors.
Moderate	› Moderate anxiety occurs when mild anxiety escalates. › Slightly reduced perception and processing of information occurs, and selective inattention can occur. › Ability to think clearly is hampered, but learning and problem-solving can still occur. › Other characteristics include concentration difficulties, tiredness, pacing, change in voice pitch, voice tremors, shakiness, and increased heart rate and respiratory rate. › The client may report somatic complaints including headaches, backache, urinary urgency and frequency, and insomnia. › The client with this type of anxiety usually benefits from the direction of others.
Severe	› Perceptual field is greatly reduced with distorted perceptions. › Learning and problem-solving do not occur. › Functioning is ineffective. › Other characteristics include confusion, feelings of impending doom, hyperventilation, tachycardia, withdrawal, loud and rapid speech, and aimless activity. › The client with severe anxiety usually is not able to take direction from others.
Panic-level	› Panic-level anxiety is characterized by markedly disturbed behavior. › The client is not able to process what is occurring in the environment and can lose touch with reality. › The client experiences extreme fright and horror. › The client experiences severe hyperactivity or flight. › Immobility can occur. › Other characteristics can include dysfunction in speech, dilated pupils, severe shakiness, severe withdrawal, inability to sleep, delusions, and hallucinations.

Patient-Centered Care

- Nursing interventions are implemented according to the level of anxiety that a client is experiencing.

NURSING INTERVENTIONS FOR THE CLIENT WITH MILD TO MODERATE LEVELS OF ANXIETY	
Nursing Intervention	Therapeutic Intent
› Use active listening to demonstrate willingness to help, and use specific communication techniques (open-ended questions, giving broad openings, exploring, and seeking clarification).	› These interventions encourage the client to express feelings, develop trust, and identify the source of the anxiety.
› Provide a calm presence, recognizing the client's distress.	› This assists the client to focus and to begin to problem-solve.
› Evaluate past coping mechanisms.	› This will assist the client to identify adaptive and nonadaptive coping mechanisms.
› Explore alternatives to problem situations.	› This intervention offers options for problem-solving.
› Encourage participation in activities, such as exercise, that can temporarily relieve feelings of inner tension.	› This provides the client with an outlet for pent-up tension, promotes endorphin release, and improves mental well-being.

NURSING INTERVENTIONS FOR THE CLIENT WITH SEVERE TO PANIC LEVELS OF ANXIETY	
Nursing Intervention	Therapeutic Intent
› Provide an environment that meets the physical and safety needs of the client. Remain with the client.	› This intervention minimizes risk to the client. The client may be unaware of the need for basic things, such as fluids, food, and sleep.
› Provide a quiet environment with minimal stimulation.	› This helps to prevent intensification of the current level of anxiety.
› Use medications and restraint, but only after less restrictive interventions have failed to decrease anxiety to safer levels.	› Medications and/or restraint may be necessary to prevent harm to the client, other clients, and providers.
› Encourage gross motor activities, such as walking and other forms of exercise.	› This provides the client with an outlet for pent-up tension, promotes endorphin release, and improves mental well-being.
› Set limits by using firm, short, and simple statements. Repetition may be necessary.	› Limit-setting can minimize risk to the client and providers. Clear, simple communication facilitates understanding.
› Direct the client to acknowledge reality and focus on what is present in the environment.	› Focusing on reality will assist with reducing the client's anxiety level.

APPLICATION EXERCISES

1. A nurse is caring for a client who smokes and has lung cancer. The client reports, "I'm coughing because I have that cold that everyone has been getting." Which of the following defense mechanisms is the client using?

    A. Reaction formation

    B. Denial

    C. Displacement

    D. Sublimation

2. A nurse is obtaining informed consent for a client who has just learned she must have a breast biopsy. The client is perspiring and pale, has a respiratory rate 30/min, and says, "I don't quite understand what you're trying to tell me." The nurse should evaluate the client's anxiety as which of the following?

    A. Mild

    B. Moderate

    C. Severe

    D. Panic

3. A nurse is caring for a client who is experiencing moderate anxiety. Which of the following is an appropriate nursing intervention when trying to give necessary information to the client?

    A. Reassure the client that everything will be okay.

    B. Use a low-pitched voice and speak slowly.

    C. Ignore the client's anxiety so that she will not be embarrassed.

    D. Demonstrate a calm manner while using simple and clear language.

4. A nurse is caring for a client who has severe anxiety. Use the ATI Active Learning Template: Basic Concept to complete this item by identifying four nursing interventions that the nurse can use to assist the client who is experiencing a severe anxiety.

APPLICATION EXERCISES KEY

1. A. INCORRECT: This is not an example of reaction formation, which is overcompensating or demonstrating the opposite behavior of what is felt.

    B. **CORRECT:** This is an example of denial, which is pretending the truth is not reality to manage the anxiety of acknowledging what is real.

    C. INCORRECT: This is not an example of displacement, which is shifting feelings related to an object, person, or situation to another less threatening object, person, or situation.

    D. INCORRECT: This is not an example of sublimation, which is dealing with unacceptable feelings or impulses by unconsciously substituting acceptable forms of expression.

    N NCLEX® Connection: Psychosocial Integrity, Mental Health Concepts

2. A. INCORRECT: In mild anxiety, the person's ability to understand information can actually increase.

    B. **CORRECT:** Moderate anxiety decreases problem-solving and can hamper one's ability to understand information. Vital signs can increase somewhat, and the person is visibly anxious.

    C. INCORRECT: Severe anxiety causes restlessness, decreased perception, and an inability to take direction.

    D. INCORRECT: During a panic attack, the person is completely distracted, unable to function, and can lose touch with reality.

    N NCLEX® Connection: Psychosocial Integrity, Crisis Intervention

3. A. INCORRECT: Providing false reassurance is not an appropriate nursing intervention.

    B. INCORRECT: Using a low-pitched voice and speaking slowly is not an appropriate nursing intervention. This is appropriate for the client who is experiencing severe to panic levels of anxiety.

    C. INCORRECT: Ignoring the client's anxiety to prevent embarrassment is not an appropriate intervention.

    D. **CORRECT:** Giving information simply and calmly will help the client grasp essential facts.

    N NCLEX® Connection: Psychosocial Integrity, Therapeutic Communication

4. *Using the ATI Active Learning Template: Basic Concept*
    - Provide an environment that meets the physical and safety needs of the client. Remain with the client.
    - Provide a quiet environment with minimal stimulation.
    - Use medications and restraint, but only after less restrictive interventions have failed to decrease anxiety to safer levels.
    - Encourage gross motor activities, such as walking and other forms of exercise.
    - Set limits by using firm, short, and simple statements. Repetition may be necessary.
    - Direct the client to acknowledge reality and focus on what is present in the environment.

    N NCLEX® Connection: Psychosocial Integrity, Behavioral Management

UNIT 1   FOUNDATIONS FOR MENTAL HEALTH NURSING

CHAPTER 5   Creating and Maintaining a Therapeutic
and Safe Environment

Overview

- Therapeutic encounters can occur in any nursing setting if a nurse is sensitive to a client's needs and uses effective communication skills.

- The therapeutic nurse-client relationship is foundational to mental health nursing care.

- The therapeutic nurse-client relationship differs from social and intimate relationships. A therapeutic nurse-client relationship is:

  ○ Purposeful and goal-directed.

  ○ Well-defined with clear boundaries.

  ○ Structured to meet the client's needs.

  ○ Characterized by an interpersonal process that is safe, confidential, reliable, and consistent.

- Milieu therapy creates an environment that is supportive, therapeutic, and safe.

  ○ Milieu therapy began as an effort to provide an environment conducive to the treatment of children who have a mental illness.

  ○ Management of the milieu refers to the management of the total environment of the mental health unit in order to provide the least amount of stress, while promoting the greatest benefit for all the clients.

  ○ The goal is that while the client is in this therapeutic environment, he will learn the tools necessary to cope adaptively, interact more effectively and appropriately, and strengthen relationship skills. Hopefully, the client will use these tools in all other aspects of his life.

  ○ The nurse participates in structuring and/or implementing aspects of the therapeutic milieu within the mental health facility.

  ○ One structure of the therapeutic milieu is regular community meetings, which include both the clients and the nursing staff.

The Therapeutic Nurse-Client Relationship

- Roles of the Nurse
  - ○ Consistently focus on the client's ideas, experiences, and feelings.
  - ○ Identify and explore the client's needs and problems.
  - ○ Discuss problem-solving alternatives with the client.
  - ○ Help to develop the client's strengths and new coping skills.
  - ○ Encourage positive behavior change in the client.
  - ○ Assist the client to develop a sense of autonomy and self-reliance.
  - ○ Portray genuineness, empathy, and a positive regard toward the client.
    - The nurse practices empathy by remaining nonjudgmental and attempting to understand the client's actions and feelings. This differs from sympathy, in which the nurse allows herself to feel the way the client does and is nontherapeutic.
- Benefits of the Therapeutic Relationship
  - ○ Therapeutic relationships contribute to the well-being of those who have a mental illness, as well as other clients, although the treatment goals will be individualized.
  - ○ These relationships take time to establish, but even time-limited therapeutic encounters can have positive outcomes.
  - ○ Therapeutic relationships have a positive impact on the success of treatment.
- Supervision by peers or the clinical team enhances the nurse's ability to examine thoughts and feelings, maintain boundaries, and continue to learn from nurse-client relationships.

FACTORS THAT POSITIVELY AFFECT THE DEVELOPMENT OF THE THERAPEUTIC RELATIONSHIP		
Nurse Factors	› Consistent approach to interaction › Adjustment of pace to client's needs › Attentive listening › Positive initial impressions	› Comfort level during the relationship › Self-awareness of own thoughts and feelings › Consistent availability
Client Factors	› Trusting attitude › Willingness to talk	› Active participation › Consistent availability

PHASES AND TASKS OF A THERAPEUTIC RELATIONSHIP	
NURSE	**CLIENT**
Orientation	
› Introduce self to the client and state purpose. › Set the contract: meeting time, place, frequency, duration, and date of termination. › Discuss confidentiality. › Build trust by establishing expectations and boundaries. › Discuss goals with the client. › Explore the client's ideas, issues, and needs. › Explore the meaning of testing behaviors. › Enforce limits on testing or other inappropriate behaviors.	› Meet with the nurse. › Agree to the contract. › Understand the limits of confidentiality. › Understand the expectations and limits of the relationship. › Participate in setting goals. › Begin to explore own thoughts, experiences, and feelings. › Explore the meaning of own behaviors.
Working	
› Maintain relationship according to the contract. › Perform ongoing data collection to plan and monitor therapeutic measures. › Facilitate the client's expression of needs and issues. › Encourage the client to problem-solve. › Promote the client's self-esteem. › Foster positive behavioral change. › Explore and deal with resistance and other defense mechanisms. › Recognize transference and countertransference issues. › Monitor and document the client's problems and goals, and contribute to replanning as necessary. › Support the client's adaptive alternatives and use of new coping skills. › Remind the client about the date of termination.	› Explore problematic areas of life. › Reconsider usual coping behaviors. › Examine own world view and self-concept. › Describe major conflicts and various defenses. › Experience intense feelings, and learn to cope with anxiety reactions. › Test new behaviors. › Begin to develop awareness of transference situations. › Try alternative solutions.
Termination	
› Provide opportunity for the client to discuss thoughts and feelings about termination and loss. › Discuss the client's previous experience with separations and loss. › Elicit the client's feelings about the therapeutic work in the nurse-client relationship. › Summarize goals and achievements. › Review memories of work in the sessions. › Express own feelings about sessions to validate the experience with the client. › Discuss ways for the client to incorporate new healthy behaviors into life. › Maintain limits of final termination.	› Discuss thoughts and feelings about termination. › Examine previous separation and loss experiences. › Explore the meaning of the therapeutic relationship. › Review goals and achievements. › Discuss plans to continue new behaviors. › Express any feelings of loss related to termination. › Make plans for the future. › Accept termination as final.

- Boundaries of the Therapeutic Relationship
  - Boundaries must be established in order to maintain a safe and professional nurse-client relationship.
  - Blurred boundaries occur if the relationship begins to meet the needs of the nurse rather than those of the client, or if the relationship becomes social rather than therapeutic.
    - Social relationship – Primary purpose is for socialization or friendship with a focus on the mutual needs of the individuals involved in the relationship.
    - Therapeutic relationship – Primary purpose is to identify the client's problems or needs and then focus on assisting the client in meeting or resolving those issues.
  - The nurse must work to maintain a consistent level of involvement with the client, to reflect on boundary issues frequently, and to maintain awareness of how behaviors can be perceived by others (clients, family members, other health team members).

TRANSFERENCE	
Description	› Transference occurs when the client views a member of the health care team as having characteristics of another person who has been significant to the client's personal life.
Example	› A client might see a nurse as being like his mother, and thus may demonstrate some of the same behaviors with the nurse as he demonstrated with his mother.
Nursing Implications	› A nurse should be aware that transference by a client is more likely to occur with a person in authority.
COUNTERTRANSFERENCE	
Description	› Countertransference occurs when a health care team member displaces characteristics of people in her past onto a client.
Example	› A nurse can feel defensive and angry with a client for no apparent reason if the client reminds her of a friend who often elicited those feelings.
Nursing Implications	› A nurse should be aware that clients who induce very strong personal feelings can become objects of countertransference.

CHARACTERISTICS OF THE THERAPEUTIC MILIEU	
Physical setting	
› Unit should be clean and orderly. › The setting should include comfortable furniture placed so that it promotes interaction, solitary spaces for reading and thinking alone, comfortable places conducive to meals, and quiet areas for sleeping.	› Color scheme and overall design should be appropriate for the client's age. › Materials used for such features as floors should be attractive, easy to clean, and safe. › Traffic-flow considerations should be conducive to client and staff movement.
Health care team member responsibilities	
› Promote independence for self-care and individual growth in clients. › Treat clients as individuals. › Allow choices for clients within the daily routine and within individual treatment plans. › Apply rules of fair treatment for all clients. › Model good social behavior for clients, such as respect for the rights of others. › Work cooperatively as a team to provide care.	› Maintain boundaries with clients. › Maintain a professional appearance and demeanor. › Promote safe and satisfying peer interactions among the clients. › Practice open communication techniques with health team members and clients. › Promote feelings of self-worth and hope for the future.
Emotional climate	
› Clients should feel safe from harm (self-harm, as well as harm from disruptive behaviors of other clients).	› Clients should feel cared for and accepted by the staff and others.

- Physical Safety
  - The nurses' station and other areas should be placed to allow for easy observation of clients by staff and access to staff by clients.
  - Special safety features, such as bathroom bars and wheelchair accessibility for clients who are disabled, should be addressed.

  - Set up the following provisions to prevent client self-harm or harm by others.
    - No access to sharp or otherwise harmful objects
    - Restriction of client access to restricted or locked areas
    - Monitoring of visitors
    - Restriction of alcohol and illegal substance access or use
    - Restriction of sexual activity among clients
    - Deterrence of elopement from facility
    - Rapid de-escalation of disruptive and potentially violent behaviors through planned interventions by trained staff
  - Seclusion rooms and restraints should be set up for safety and used only after all less-restrictive measures have been exhausted. When used, facility policies and procedures must be followed.
  - Plan for safe access to recreational areas, occupational therapy, and meeting rooms.

- ○ Teach fire, evacuation, and other safety rules to all staff.
  - ▪ Have clear plans for keeping clients and staff safe in emergencies.
  - ▪ Maintain staff skills, such as cardiopulmonary resuscitation.
- ○ Considerations of room assignments on a 24-hr care unit should include:
  - ▪ Personalities of each roommate.
  - ▪ The likelihood of nighttime disruptions for a roommate if one client has difficulty sleeping.
  - ▪ Mental health and medical diagnoses, such as how two clients who have severe paranoia might interact with each other.
- ○ Activities within the therapeutic milieu are structured and include time for the following.

  - ▪ Community meetings
    - ▫ The community meeting on the mental health unit should enhance the emotional climate of the therapeutic milieu by promoting:
      - ▸ Interaction and communication between staff and clients.
      - ▸ Decision-making skills of clients.
      - ▸ A feeling of self-worth among clients.
      - ▸ Discussions of common unit objectives, such as encouraging clients to meet treatment goals and plan for discharge.
      - ▸ Discussion of issues of concern to all members of the unit, including common problems, future activities, and the introduction of new clients to the unit.
      - ▸ Meetings may be structured so that they are client-led with decisions made by the group as a whole.
  - ▪ Individual therapy – scheduled sessions with a mental health provider to address specific mental health concerns, such as depression
  - ▪ Group therapy – scheduled sessions for a group of clients to address common mental health issues, such as substance use disorder
  - ▪ Psychoeducational groups – based on a client's level of functioning and personal needs, such as adverse effects of medication
  - ▪ Recreational activities, such as a game or a community outing
  - ▪ Unstructured, flexible time that includes opportunities for the nurse and other staff to observe clients as they interact spontaneously within the milieu

APPLICATION EXERCISES

1. A nurse is talking with a client who is at risk for suicide following the death of his spouse. Which of the following statements by the nurse is appropriate?

    A. "I feel very sorry for the loneliness you must be experiencing."

    B. "Suicide is not the appropriate way to cope with loss."

    C. "Losing someone close to you must be very upsetting."

    D. "I know how difficult it is to lose a loved one."

2. A nurse is in the working phase of a therapeutic relationship with a client who has methamphetamine use disorder. Which of the following indicates transference behavior?

    A. The client asks the nurse whether she will go out to dinner with him.

    B. The client accuses the nurse of telling him what to do just like his ex-girlfriend.

    C. The client reminds the nurse of a friend who died from a substance overdose.

    D. The client becomes angry and threatens harm to himself.

3. A nurse is discussing the characteristics of a nurse-client relationship with a newly licensed nurse. Which of the following are appropriate to include in the discussion? (Select all that apply.)

    _____ A. The needs of both participants are met.

    _____ B. An emotional commitment exists between the participants.

    _____ C. It is goal-directed.

    _____ D. Behavioral change is encouraged.

    _____ E. A termination date is established.

4. A nurse is assisting with planning care for the termination phase of a nurse-client relationship. Which of the following actions is appropriate to include in the plan of care?

    A. Discussing ways to use new behaviors

    B. Practicing new problem-solving skills

    C. Developing goals

    D. Establishing boundaries

5. A nurse is orienting a new client to a mental health unit. When explaining the unit's community meetings, which of the following statements by the nurse is appropriate?

    A. "You and a group of other clients will meet to discuss your treatment plans."

    B. "Community meetings have a specific agenda that is established by staff."

    C. "You and the other clients will meet with staff to discuss common problems."

    D. "Community meetings are an excellent opportunity to explore your personal mental health issues."

6. A nurse is discussing a therapeutic milieu during the orientation of a newly hired nurse. Use the ATI Active Learning Template: Basic Concept to complete this item to include the following sections:

    A. Underlying Principles: Identify at least five responsibilities of the health care team to maintain a therapeutic milieu.

    B. Nursing Interventions: Identify at least four interventions to prevent client self-harm or harm by others.

APPLICATION EXERCISES KEY

1. A. INCORRECT: This statement focuses on the nurse's feelings and is sympathetic rather than empathetic.

    B. INCORRECT: This statement implies judgment and is therefore not an empathetic or therapeutic response.

    C. **CORRECT:** This statement is an empathetic response that attempts to understand the client's feelings.

    D. INCORRECT: This statement focuses on the nurse's experiences rather than the client's and is therefore not therapeutic.

    Ⓝ NCLEX® Connection: Psychosocial Integrity, Therapeutic Communication

2. A. INCORRECT: This indicates the need to discuss boundaries but does not indicate transference.

    B. **CORRECT:** When a client views the nurse as having characteristics of another person who has been significant to his personal life, such as his ex-girlfriend, this indicates transference.

    C. INCORRECT: This indicates countertransference rather than transference.

    D. INCORRECT: This indicates the need for safety intervention but does not indicate transference.

    Ⓝ NCLEX® Connection: Psychosocial Integrity, Therapeutic Communication

3. A. INCORRECT: A therapeutic nurse-client relationship focuses on the needs of the client.

    B. INCORRECT: An emotional commitment between the participants is characteristic of an intimate or social relationship rather than one that is therapeutic.

    C. **CORRECT:** A therapeutic nurse-client relationship is goal-directed.

    D. **CORRECT:** A therapeutic nurse-client relationship encourages positive behavioral change.

    E. **CORRECT:** A therapeutic nurse-client relationship has an established termination date.

    Ⓝ NCLEX® Connection: Psychosocial Integrity, Therapeutic Communication

4. A. **CORRECT:** Discussing ways for the client to incorporate new healthy behaviors into life is an appropriate task for the termination phase.

    B. INCORRECT: Practicing new problem-solving skills is an appropriate task for the working phase.

    C. INCORRECT: Developing goals is an appropriate task for the orientation phase.

    D. INCORRECT: Establishing boundaries is an appropriate task for the orientation phase.

    Ⓝ NCLEX® Connection: Psychosocial Integrity, Therapeutic Communication

5. A. INCORRECT: Individual treatment plans are discussed during individual therapy rather than a community meeting.

    B. INCORRECT: Community meetings can be structured so that they are client-led with decisions made by the group as a whole.

    C. **CORRECT:** Community meetings are an opportunity for clients to discuss common problems or issues affecting all members of the unit.

    D. INCORRECT: Personal mental health issues are discussed during individual therapy rather than a community meeting.

    (N) NCLEX® Connection: Psychosocial Integrity, Therapeutic Environment

6. *Using ATI Active Learning Template: Basic Concept*

    A. Underlying Principles

    • Promote independence for self-care and individual growth.

    • Treat clients as individuals.

    • Allow choices for clients within the daily routine and treatment plan.

    • Apply rules of fair treatment for all clients.

    • Model good social behavior.

    • Work cooperatively as a team to provide care.

    • Maintain boundaries with clients.

    • Maintain a professional appearance and demeanor.

    • Promote safe and satisfying peer interactions among clients.

    • Practice open communication techniques with health team members and clients.

    • Promote feelings of self-worth and hope for the future.

    B. Nursing Interventions

    • Prevent access to sharp or harmful objects.

    • Restrict client access to restricted or locked areas.

    • Monitor visitors.

    • Restrict alcohol and illegal substance access and use.

    • Restrict sexual activity among clients.

    • Deter elopement from facility.

    • Provide rapid de-escalation of disruptive and potentially violent behaviors.

    • Be aware of facility policies and procedures for seclusion or restraints.

    • Provide safe access to recreational areas, therapy, and meeting rooms.

    (N) NCLEX® Connection: Psychosocial Integrity, Therapeutic Environment

UNIT 1   FOUNDATIONS FOR MENTAL HEALTH NURSING

CHAPTER 6   Diverse Practice Settings

Overview

- Acute Care Settings for Mental Health Care
  - This setting provides intensive treatment and supervision in locked units for clients who have severe mental illness.
  - Care in these facilities helps stabilize mental illness symptoms and promotes the clients' return to the community.
  - Staff is made up of an interprofessional team.
  - Facilities can be privately owned, with payment provided by private funds or insurance.
  - Facilities also can be state-owned, with much of the funding provided for indigent clients. State-run facilities also often provide full-time acute care for forensic clients (those in a correctional setting) with severe mental illness.
  - Case management programs assist with client transition to a community setting after discharge from the acute care facility.
- Community Settings for Mental Health Care
  - Primary care is provided in community-based settings, which include clinics, schools and day-care centers, partial hospitalization programs, drug and alcohol treatment facilities, forensic settings, psychosocial rehabilitation programs, telephone crisis counseling centers, and home health care.
  - Nurses working in community care programs help to stabilize or improve clients' mental functioning within a community. They also reinforce teaching, provide support, and make referrals in order to promote positive social activities.
  - Nursing interventions in community settings provide for primary treatment as well as primary, secondary, and tertiary prevention of mental illness.
- Forensic Nursing
  - Forensic nursing is a combination of biophysical education and forensic science. The registered nurses use scientific investigation, collection of evidence, analysis, prevention, and treatment of trauma and/or death of perpetrators and victims of violence, abuse, and traumatic accidents.
- In all settings, nurses are advocates for clients who have mental illness. Referral of clients and their families to organizations and agencies that provide additional resources can provide significant support to individuals. For example, the National Alliance on Mental Illness (NAMI) is a grassroots organization with the goals of improving the quality of life for people who have mental illness and providing research to better treat or eradicate mental illness. For more information, go to www.nami.org.

History of Mental Health Care in the United States

- Most clients who had severe mental illness were treated solely in acute care inpatient facilities before the middle of the 20th century.

- Congress passed a series of acts in 1946, 1955, and 1963 in response to the appalling condition of facilities for the mentally ill. This began a trend to deinstitutionalize mental health care.

- Clients who had lived in acute care mental health facilities for many years were discharged into the community at a time when community mental health facilities often were unprepared to deal with this influx.

- The concept of the case manager was introduced around 1970 to meet the individual needs of clients in a mental health setting.

- Managed care through health maintenance organizations (HMOs), preferred provider organizations (PPOs), and others began limiting hospital stays for clients in a general medical setting starting around 1980.

  ○ Managed Behavioral Healthcare Organizations (MBHOs) later developed to coordinate care and limit stays in acute care facilities for clients needing mental health care.

  ○ This began the trend to develop a continuum of acute care facilities and community mental health facilities to provide for all levels of behavioral health care needs.

  ○ Complete and accurate documentation of client needs and progress by nurses and other health care professionals is needed to ensure quality care for each client.

- Factors that will affect the future of mental health care include the following.

  ○ An increase in the aging population

  ○ An increase in cultural diversity within the United States

  ○ The expansion of technology, which may provide new settings for client care, as well as new ways to treat mental illness more effectively

Client Care in Acute Mental Health Care Settings

- Criteria to justify admission to an acute care facility include:

  ○ A clear risk of the client's danger to self or others

  ○ The failure of community-based treatment

  ○ A dangerous decline in the mental health status of a client undergoing long-term treatment

  ○ A client having a medical need in addition to a mental illness

- Goals of acute mental health treatment include:

  ○ Prevention of the client harming self or others

  ○ Stabilizing mental health crises

  ○ Return of clients who are severally ill to some type of community care

- Interprofessional team members in acute care include nurses, mental health technicians (who perform duties similar to assistive personnel in other health care facilities), psychologists, psychiatrists, other general health care providers, social workers, counselors, occupational and other specialty therapists, and pharmacists.

  ○ The interprofessional team has the primary responsibility of planning and monitoring individualized treatment plans or clinical pathways of care, depending on the philosophy and policy of the facility.

  ○ Plans for discharge to home or to a community facility begin from the time of admission and continue with the implementation of the initial treatment plan or clinical pathway.

  ○ Nurses in acute care mental health facilities use the nursing process and a holistic approach to provide care. Nursing roles include the following.

    ▪ Participating in client activities and therapeutic milieu

    ▪ Ensuring safe administration and monitoring of all client medications

    ▪ Reinforcement of client teaching

    ▪ Documentation of the client's response to care

    ▪ Participating in crises management

Client Care In Community Health Settings

- Nurses are responsible for identifying community resources.

- Intensive outpatient programs promote community reintegration for clients.

- Three levels of prevention are used by nurses when implementing community care interventions/education.

LEVEL OF PREVENTION	EXAMPLES OF INTERVENTIONS
› Primary prevention promotes health and prevents mental health problems from occurring.	› A nurse leads a group for parents of toddlers, discussing normal toddler behavior and ways to promote healthy development.
› Secondary prevention focuses on early detection of mental illness.	› A nurse provides assistance for screening of parents of children who have developmental disorders.
› Tertiary prevention focuses on rehabilitation and prevention of further problems in clients previously diagnosed.	› A nurse participates in a support group for clients who have completed a substance use disorder program.

- Community-based mental health programs are a continuum of mental health agencies with varying treatment intensity levels to allow clients to remain safe in the least restrictive environment possible.

COMMUNITY-BASED MENTAL HEALTH PROGRAMS

Partial hospitalization programs

› These programs provide intense short-term treatment for clients who are well enough to go home every night and who have a responsible person at home to provide support and a safe environment.

› Certain detoxification programs are a specialized form of partial hospitalization for clients who require medical supervision, stress management, substance use disorder counseling, and relapse prevention.

Assertive community treatment (ACT)

› This includes nontraditional case management and treatment by an interprofessional team for clients who have severe mental illness and are noncompliant with traditional treatment.

› ACT helps reduce reoccurrences of hospitalizations and provides crisis intervention, assistance with independent living, and information regarding resources for necessary support services.

Community mental health centers

› These facilities provide a variety of services for a wide range of community clients.
  » Educational groups
  » Medication dispensing programs
  » Individual counseling programs

Psychosocial rehabilitation programs

› These programs provide a structured range of programs for clients in a mental health setting.
  » Residential services
  » Day programs for older adults

Home care

› Home care provides mental health assessment, interventions, and family support in the client's home. This is implemented most often for children, older adults, and clients who have other medical conditions.

Roles of Nurses in Diverse Mental Health Practice Settings

REGISTERED NURSE	PRACTICAL NURSE	ADVANCED PRACTICE NURSE
› Educational preparation: diploma, associate degree, or baccalaureate degree in nursing, with additional on-the-job training and continuing education in mental health care.	› Educational preparation: typically completion of an associate's degree through a vocational school, technical school, or community college.	› Educational preparation: advanced nursing degree in behavioral health (master's degree, doctorate, nurse practitioner, or clinical nurse specialist).
› May work in either an acute care or community-based facility.	› May work in either an acute care or community-based facility.	› May work independently, often supervising individuals or groups in either an acute care or community-based setting.
› Functions within a facility using the nursing process to provide care and treatment, such as medication.	› Functions within a facility using the nursing process to provide care and treatment such as medication.	› May have prescription privileges and is able to independently recommend interventions.
› Manages care for a group of clients within a unit of the facility.	› Participates in the care for a group of clients within a unit of the facility.	› May manage and administrate the care for an entire facility.

APPLICATION EXERCISES

1. A nurse is working in a community mental health facility. Which of the following services are appropriate for clients to receive? (Select all that apply).

_____ A. Educational groups

_____ B. Medication dispensing programs

_____ C. Individual counseling programs

_____ D. Detoxification programs

_____ E. Crisis intervention

2. A nurse is caring for several clients who are attending community-based mental health programs. Which of the following clients should the nurse plan to visit first?

   A. A client who recently burned her arm while using a hot iron at home

   B. A client who requests that her antipsychotic medication be changed due to some new side effects

   C. A client who says he is hearing a voice that tells him he is not worthy of living anymore

   D. A client who tells the nurse he experienced symptoms of severe anxiety before and during a job interview

3. A nurse is working on promotion of healthy coping skills with older adult clients who all previously had been hospitalized for severe depression and are now in a residential care facility. The nurse should recognize that this is an example of which of the following?

   A. Primary prevention

   B. Secondary prevention

   C. Tertiary prevention

   D. Mental status examination

4. A nurse is caring for a group of clients. Which of the following clients should a nurse consider for referral to an assertive community treatment (ACT) group?

    A. A client in an acute care mental health facility who has fallen several times while running down the hallway

    B. A client who lives at home and keeps "forgetting" to come in for his monthly antipsychotic injection for schizophrenia

    C. A client in a day treatment program who says he is becoming more anxious during group therapy

    D. A client in a weekly grief support group who says she still misses her husband who has been dead for 3 months

5. A nurse in an acute mental health facility is caring for a client who has a severe mental illness and soon will be ready for discharge but still requires supervision much of the time. The client's partner works all day but is home by late afternoon. Which of the following should the nurse suggest as appropriate follow-up care?

    A. Receiving daily care from a home health aide

    B. Having a weekly visit from a nurse case worker

    C. Attending a partial hospitalization program

    D. Visiting a community mental health center on a daily basis

6. A nurse is assisting an RN with an in-service education program regarding acute mental health treatment for a group of newly licensed nurses. What should the nurse include in this presentation? Use the ATI Active Learning Template: Basic Concept to complete this item to include the following:

    A. Related Content: Identify two criteria for admitting a client to a mental health facility.

    B. Underlying Principles: Describe two concepts of mental health treatment.

    C. Nursing Interventions: Describe two nursing interventions.

APPLICATION EXERCISES KEY

1. A. **CORRECT:** Educational groups are services provided in a community mental health facility.

    B. **CORRECT:** Medication dispensing programs are services provided in a community mental health facility.

    C. **CORRECT:** Individual counseling programs are services provided in a community mental health facility.

    D. INCORRECT: Detoxification programs are services provided in a partial hospitalization program.

    E. INCORRECT: Crisis intervention is offered in an assertive community treatment (ACT) program.

    (N) NCLEX® Connection: Coordinated Care, Referral Process

2. A. INCORRECT: This client has needs that should be met, but is not as high a priority as the client at risk for self-injury.

    B. INCORRECT: This client has needs that should be met, but is not as high a priority as the client at risk for self-injury.

    C. **CORRECT:** A client who hears a voice telling him he is not worthy is at greatest risk for self-harm, and the nurse should visit this client first.

    D. INCORRECT: This client has needs that should be met, but is not as high a priority as the client at risk for self-injury.

    (N) NCLEX® Connection: Coordinated Care, Establishing Priorities

3. A. INCORRECT: Primary prevention deals with preventing the initial onset of a mental health problem.

    B. INCORRECT: Secondary prevention deals with early detection of disease.

    C. **CORRECT:** Tertiary prevention deals with prevention of further problems in clients already diagnosed with mental illness.

    D. INCORRECT: The mental status examination is a tool that the nurse could use to collect data regarding a client's problem, but it is not a type of prevention.

    (N) NCLEX® Connection: Psychosocial Integrity, Coping Mechanisms

4. A. INCORRECT: A client in acute care who has been running and falling should be helped by the treatment team on her unit.

    B. **CORRECT:** An ACT group works with clients who are nonadherent with traditional therapy, such as the client in a home setting who keeps "forgetting" his injection.

    C. INCORRECT: A client who has anxiety might be referred to his counselor or mental health provider.

    D. INCORRECT: A client who is grieving for her husband who died 3 months ago is currently involved in an appropriate intervention.

    N NCLEX® Connection: Coordinated Care, Referral Process

5. A. INCORRECT: Daily care provided by a home health aide will not provide adequate supervision for this client.

    B. INCORRECT: Weekly visits from a case worker will not provide adequate care and supervision for this client.

    C. **CORRECT:** A partial hospitalization program can provide treatment during the day while allowing the client to spend nights at home, as long as a responsible family member is present.

    D. INCORRECT: A weekly visit from a nurse case worker will not provide adequate care and supervision for this client.

    N NCLEX® Connection: Coordinated Care, Referral Process

6. *Using the ATI Active Learning Template: Basic Concept*

    A. Related Content
        - Clear risk of the client's danger to self and others
        - Failure of community based treatment
        - A dangerous decline in the mental health status of a client undergoing long-term treatment
        - A client having a medical need in addition to a mental illness

    B. Underlying Principles
        - Goals of acute mental health treatment
            - Prevention of the client harming self or others
            - Stabilizing mental health crises
            - Return of clients who are severally ill to some type of community care
        - Interprofessional team members in acute care include nurses, mental health technicians, psychologists, psychiatrists, other general health care providers, social workers, counselors, occupational and other specialty therapists, and pharmacists.

    C. Nursing Interventions
        - Who: The interprofessional team members' primary responsibility is planning and monitoring individualized treatment plans or clinical pathways of care.
        - When: Plans for discharge to home or to a community facility begin from the time of admission.
        - How: Nursing roles include participating in client activities and therapeutic milieu.
            - Ensuring safe administration and monitoring of client medications.
            - Assisting with implementation of individual client treatment plans, including client teaching.
            - Documentation of the client's response to care.
            - Participating in crisis management.

    Ⓝ NCLEX® Connection: Psychosocial Integrity, Mental Health Concepts

UNIT 2   ## Traditional Nonpharmacological Therapies

CHAPTERS

› Psychoanalysis, Psychotherapy, and Behavioral Therapies
› Group and Family Therapy
› Stress Management
› Brain Stimulation Therapies

NCLEX® CONNECTIONS

When reviewing the chapters in this unit, keep in mind the relevant sections of the NCLEX® outline, in particular:

Client Needs: Psychosocial Integrity

› Relevant topics/tasks include:
  » Behavioral Management
    › Participate in client group sessions.
  » Therapeutic Communication
    › Provide emotional support to the client and family.
  » Mental Health Concepts
    › Recognize the client's use of defense mechanisms.
  » Stress Management
    › Implement measures to reduce environmental stressors.
  » Support Systems
    › Identity the client's support systems and resources.

Client Needs: Reduction of Risk Potential

› Relevant topics/tasks include:
  » Potential for Complications of Diagnostic Tests/Treatments/Procedures
    › Provide care for the client receiving electroconvulsive therapy.

chapter 7

Overview

- Psychoanalysis, psychotherapy, and behavioral therapies are approaches to addressing mental health issues using various methods and theoretical bases.
- Nurses working in mental health settings need to be familiar with the methods that are part of these approaches and their application in practice.

Psychoanalysis

- Classical psychoanalysis is a therapeutic process of determining unconscious thoughts and feelings, and resolving conflict by talking to a psychoanalyst. Clients attend many sessions over the course of months to years.
  - Due to the length of psychoanalytic therapy and health insurance constraints, classical psychoanalysis is less likely to be the sole therapy of choice.
  - Psychoanalysis was first developed by Sigmund Freud to resolve internal conflicts which, he contended, always occur from early childhood experiences.
  - Past relationships are a common focus for therapy.
- Therapeutic tools
  - Free association, which is the spontaneous, uncensored verbalization of whatever comes to a client's mind
  - Dream analysis and interpretation
  - Transference, which includes feelings that the client has developed toward the therapist in relation to similar feelings toward significant persons in the client's early childhood
  - Use of defense mechanisms
- Psychotherapy involves more verbal therapist-to-client interaction than classic psychoanalysis.
  - The client and the therapist develop a trusting relationship to explore the client's problems.
  - Psychodynamic psychotherapy employs the same tools as psychoanalysis. But it focuses more on the client's present state, rather than his early life.
  - Interpersonal psychotherapy (IPT) assists clients in addressing specific problems. It can improve interpersonal relationships, communication, role-relationship, and bereavement.
  - Cognitive therapy is based on the cognitive model, which focuses on individual thoughts and behaviors to solve current problems. It treats depression, anxiety, eating disorders, and other issues that can improve by changing a client's attitude toward life experiences.

- ○ Behavioral Therapy

  - In protest of Freud's psychoanalytic theory, behavioral theorists such as Ivan Pavlov, John B. Watson, and B.F. Skinner thought that changing behavior was the key to treating problems such as anxiety or depressive disorders.

  - Behavioral therapy is based on the theory that behavior is learned and has consequences. Abnormal behavior results from an attempt to avoid painful feelings. Changing abnormal or maladaptive behavior can occur without the need for insight into the underlying cause of the behavior.

  - Behavioral therapies show clients ways to decrease anxiety or avoidant behavior and give clients an opportunity to practice techniques.

  - Behavioral therapy has been used successfully to treat clients who have phobias, substance use or addictive disorders, and other issues.

- ○ Cognitive-behavioral therapy uses both a cognitive and behavioral approach to assist a client with anxiety management.

  - Dialectical behavior therapy is a cognitive-behavioral therapy for clients who have a personality disorder and exhibit self-injurious behavior. This therapy focuses on gradual behavior changes and provides acceptance and validation for these clients.

Use of Cognitive Therapy

- • Cognitive Reframing

  - ○ Changing cognitive distortions can decrease anxiety. Cognitive reframing assists clients to identify negative thoughts that produce anxiety, examine the cause, and develop supportive ideas that replace negative self-talk. For example, a client who has a depressive disorder may say he is "a bad person who has never done anything good" in his life. Through therapy, this client may change his thinking to realize that he may have made some bad choices, but that he is not "a bad person."

  - Priority restructuring – Assists clients to identify what requires priority, such as devoting energy to pleasurable activities.

  - Journal keeping – Helps clients write down stressful thoughts and has a positive effect on well-being.

  - Assertiveness training – Educates clients to express feelings, and solve problems in a nonaggressive manner.

  - Monitoring thoughts – Helps clients to be aware of negative thinking.

Types and Uses of Behavioral Therapy

MODELING	
Definition	› A therapist or others serve as role models for a client, who imitates this modeling to improve behavior.
Use in Mental Health Nursing	› Modeling can occur in the acute care milieu to help clients improve interpersonal skills. The therapist demonstrates appropriate behavior in a stressful situation with the goal of having the client imitate the behavior.

OPERANT CONDITIONING	
Definition	› The client receives positive rewards for positive behavior (positive reinforcement).
Use in Mental Health Nursing	› As an example: a client receives tokens for good behavior, and he can exchange them for a privilege or other items.

SYSTEMATIC DESENSITIZATION	
Definition	› This therapy is the planned, progressive, or graduated exposure to anxiety-provoking stimuli in real-life situations, or by imagining events that cause anxiety. During exposure, the client uses relaxation techniques to suppress anxiety response.
Use in Mental Health Nursing	› Systematic desensitization begins with the client mastering relaxation techniques. Then, the client is exposed to increasing levels of the anxiety-producing stimulus (either imagined or real) and uses relaxation to overcome anxiety. The client is then able to tolerate a greater and greater level of the stimulus until anxiety no longer interferes with functioning.

AVERSION THERAPY	
Definition	› Pairing of a maladaptive behavior with a punishment or unpleasant stimuli to promote a change in the behavior.
Use in Mental Health Nursing	› A therapist or treatment team can use unpleasant stimuli, such as bitter taste or mild electric shock, as punishment for behaviors such as alcohol use disorder, violence, self-mutilation, and thumb-sucking.

MEDITATION, GUIDED IMAGERY, DIAPHRAGMATIC BREATHING, MUSCLE RELAXATION, AND BIOFEEDBACK	
Definition	› This therapy uses various techniques to control pain, tension, and anxiety.
Use in Mental Health Nursing	› As an example, a nurse can provide instructions on diaphragmatic breathing to a client having a panic attack, or to a female client in labor.

- Other techniques
  - Flooding – Exposing a client, while in the company of a therapist, to a great deal of an undesirable stimulus in an attempt to turn off the anxiety response.
  - Response prevention – Preventing a client from performing a compulsive behavior with the intent that anxiety will diminish.
  - Thought stopping – Instructing a client, when negative thoughts or compulsive behaviors arise, to say or shout, "stop," and substitute a positive thought. The goal over time is for the client to use the command silently.

APPLICATION EXERCISES

1. A nurse is reinforcing teaching with a client who has an anxiety disorder and is scheduled to begin classical psychoanalysis. Which of the following client statements indicates an understanding of this form of therapy?

    A. "Even if my anxiety improves, I will need to continue this therapy for 6 weeks."

    B. "The therapist will focus on my past relationships during our sessions."

    C. "Psychoanalysis will help me reduce my anxiety by changing my behaviors."

    D. "This therapy will address my conscious feelings about stressful experiences."

2. A nurse is discussing free association as a therapeutic tool with a client who has major depressive disorder. Which of the following client statements indicates understanding of this technique?

    A. "I will write down my dreams as soon as I wake up."

    B. "I may begin to associate my therapist with important people in my life."

    C. "I can learn to express myself in a nonaggressive manner."

    D. "I should say the first thing that comes to my mind."

3. A nurse is assisting an RN with preparing to implement cognitive reframing techniques for a client who has an anxiety disorder. Which of the following are appropriate to include in the plan of care? (Select all that apply.)

    _____ A. Priority restructuring

    _____ B. Monitoring thoughts

    _____ C. Diaphragmatic breathing

    _____ D. Journal keeping

    _____ E. Meditation

4. A nurse is caring for a client who has a prescription for disulfiram (Antabuse) for the treatment of his alcohol use disorder. The nurse informs the client that this medication can cause nausea and vomiting if he drinks alcohol. This form of treatment is an example of which of the following?

    A. Aversion therapy

    B. Flooding

    C. Biofeedback

    D. Dialectical behavior therapy

5. A nurse is assisting with systematic desensitization for a client who has an extreme fear of elevators. Which of the following is appropriate when implementing this form of therapy?

    A. Demonstrate riding in an elevator, and then ask the client to imitate the behavior.

    B. Advise the client to say "stop" out loud every time he begins to feel an anxiety response related to an elevator.

    C. Gradually expose the client to an elevator while practicing relaxation techniques.

    D. Stay with the client in an elevator until his anxiety response diminishes.

6. A nurse working in an acute mental health unit is caring for a client who has a personality disorder. The client refuses to attend group meetings and will not speak to other clients or attend unit activities. The client enjoys visiting with staff, and requests daily to take a walk outside with a staff member. The provider prescribes behavioral therapy with operant conditioning. Use the ATI Active Learning Template: Therapeutic Procedure to complete this item to include the following sections:

    A. Description of Procedure: Discuss behavioral therapy and operant conditioning.

    B. Nursing Actions: Identify an appropriate nursing action to implement operant conditioning with this client.

APPLICATION EXERCISES KEY

1. A. INCORRECT: Classical psychoanalysis is a therapeutic process that requires many sessions over months to years.

   B. **CORRECT:** Classical psychoanalysis places a common focus on past relationships to identify the cause of the anxiety disorder.

   C. INCORRECT: Classical psychoanalysis focuses on identifying and resolving the cause of the anxiety rather than changing behavior.

   D. INCORRECT: Classical psychoanalysis assesses unconscious, rather than conscious, thoughts and feelings.

   Ⓝ NCLEX® Connection: Psychosocial Integrity, Therapeutic Communication

2. A. INCORRECT: Dream analysis and interpretation are therapeutic tools. However, they are not an example of free association.

   B. INCORRECT: Associating the therapist with significant persons in the client's life is an example of transference, rather than free association.

   C. INCORRECT: Learning to express feelings and solve problems in a nonaggressive manner is an example of assertiveness training, rather than free association.

   D. **CORRECT:** Free association is the spontaneous, uncensored verbalization of whatever comes to a client's mind.

   Ⓝ NCLEX® Connection: Psychosocial Integrity, Therapeutic Communication

3. A. **CORRECT:** Priority restructuring is a cognitive reframing technique.

   B. **CORRECT:** Monitoring thoughts is a cognitive reframing technique.

   C. INCORRECT: Diaphragmatic breathing is a form of behavioral therapy, rather than a cognitive reframing technique.

   D. **CORRECT:** Journal keeping is a cognitive reframing technique.

   E. INCORRECT: Meditation is a form of behavioral therapy, rather than a cognitive reframing technique.

   Ⓝ NCLEX® Connection: Psychosocial Integrity, Behavioral Management

4.   A.   **CORRECT:** Aversion therapy pairs a maladaptive behavior with unpleasant stimuli to promote a change in behavior.

     B.   INCORRECT: Flooding is planned exposure to an undesirable stimulus in an attempt to turn off the anxiety response.

     C.   INCORRECT: Biofeedback is a behavioral therapy to control pain, tension, and anxiety.

     D.   INCORRECT: Dialectical behavior therapy is a cognitive-behavioral therapy for clients who have a personality disorder and exhibit self-injurious behavior.

     Ⓝ NCLEX® Connection: Psychosocial Integrity, Chemical and Other Dependencies

5.   A.   INCORRECT: Demonstration followed by client imitation of the behavior is an example of modeling, rather than systematic desensitization.

     B.   INCORRECT: Instructing a client to say "stop" when anxiety occurs is an example of thought stopping, rather than systematic desensitization.

     C.   **CORRECT:** Systematic desensitization is the planned, progressive exposure to anxiety-provoking stimuli. During this exposure, relaxation techniques suppress the anxiety response.

     D.   INCORRECT: Exposing the client to a great deal of an undesirable stimulus in an attempt to turn off the anxiety response is an example of flooding, rather than systematic desensitization.

     Ⓝ NCLEX® Connection: Psychosocial Integrity, Behavioral Management

6.   *Using the ATI Active Learning Template: Therapeutic Procedure*

     A. Description of Procedure
        • Behavioral therapy is based on the theory that behavior is learned and has consequences. These therapies educate clients on ways to decrease anxiety or avoidant behavior and give clients an opportunity to practice techniques.
        • Operant conditioning provides the client with positive rewards for positive behavior.

     B. Nursing Actions
        • The nurse will use tokens, or something similar, to reward the client for a positive change in behavior. The client can use these tokens for larger rewards, such as a walk outside with a staff member.
        • The nurse will provide positive feedback and encouragement for a positive change in behavior.

     Ⓝ NCLEX® Connection: Psychosocial Integrity, Behavioral Management

chapter 8

Overview

- Therapy is an intensive treatment that involves open therapeutic communication with participants who are willing to take part in therapy.
- Although individual therapy is an important treatment for mental illness, group and family therapies are also a part of the treatment plan for many clients in a mental health setting.
- Leaders guide group and family therapy, and they can employ various leadership styles.
  - Democratic – This style supports group interaction and decision-making to solve problems.
  - Laissez-faire – The group process progresses without any attempt by the leader to control the direction.
  - Autocratic – The leader completely controls the direction and structure of the group without allowing group interaction or decision making to solve problems.
- Examples of group therapy include stress management, substance use disorders, medication education, understanding mental illness, and dual diagnosis groups.

Group Therapy

- Group process is the verbal and nonverbal communication that occurs within the group during group sessions.
- Group norm is the way the group behaves during sessions. Over time, it provides structure for the group. For example, a group norm could be that members raise their hand to be recognized by the leader before they speak. Another norm could be that all members sit in the same places for each session.
- Hidden agenda – Some group members (or the leader) might have goals different from the stated group goals that can disrupt group processes. For example, three members might try to embarrass another member whom they dislike.
- A subgroup is a small number of people within a larger group who function separately from the group.
- Groups can be open (new members join as old members leave) or closed (no new members join after formation of the group).
- A homogenous group is one in which all members share a certain chosen characteristic, such as diagnosis or gender. Membership of heterogeneous groups is not based on a shared chosen personal characteristic. An example of a heterogeneous group is all clients on a unit, including a mixture of males and females who have a wide range of diagnoses.
- All therapy sessions need to include:
  - The use of open and clear communication.
  - Cohesiveness and guidelines for the therapy session.
  - Direction toward a particular goal.
  - Opportunities for the development of interpersonal skills, resolution of personal and family issues, and the development of appropriate, satisfying relationships.

- ○ Encouragement of the client to maximize positive interactions, feel empowered to make decisions, and strengthen feelings of self-worth.
- ○ Communication regarding respect among all members.
- ○ Support, as well as education regarding things such as available community resources for support.
- Group therapy goals
  - ○ Sharing of common feelings and concerns
  - ○ Sharing of stories and experiences
  - ○ Diminishing feelings of isolation
  - ○ Creating a community of healing and restoration
  - ○ Providing a more cost-effective environment than that of individual therapy
- Varying age groups can use group therapy

  - ○ Children – It is in the form of play while talking about a common experience.
  - ○ Adolescent – It is especially valuable, as this age group typically has strong peer relationships.
  - ○ Older adult – It helps with socialization and sharing of memories.

PHASES OF GROUP DEVELOPMENT	
INITIAL PHASE	
Primary Focus	› Define the purpose and goals of the group.
Responsibilities	› The group leader sets a tone of respect, trust, and confidentiality among members.
	› Members get to know each other and the group leader.
	› There's a discussion about termination.
WORKING PHASE	
Primary Focus	› Promote problem-solving skills to facilitate behavioral changes. Power and control issues can dominate in this phase.
Responsibilities	› The group leader uses therapeutic communication to encourage group work toward meeting goals.
	› Members take informal roles within the group, which can interfere with, or favor, group progress toward goals.
TERMINATION PHASE	
Primary Focus	› This marks the end of group sessions.
Responsibilities	› Group members discuss termination issues.
	› The leader summarizes work of the group and individual contributions.

- Members of a group can take on any of a number of roles
  - ○ Maintenance roles – Members who take on these roles tend to help maintain the purpose and process of the group. For example, the harmonizer attempts to prevent conflict in the group.
  - ○ Task roles – Members take on various tasks within the group process. An example of a task role is the recorder, who takes notes and records what occurs during each session.
  - ○ Individual roles – These roles tend to prevent teamwork, because individuals take on roles to promote their own agenda. Examples include the dominator, who tries to control other members, and the recognition seeker, who boasts about personal achievements.

- Group characteristics can vary depending on the health care setting.
  - Groups in an acute mental health setting – Members can vary on a daily basis, and the focus of the group is on relief. Unit activities will directly impact the group, and the leader must provide a higher level of structure.
  - Groups in an outpatient setting – Members are often consistent, the focus of the group is on growth, external influences are limited, and the leader can allow members an opportunity in determining the group's direction.

Characteristics of Families

- Families can have healthy or dysfunctional characteristics in one or more areas of functioning.

AREAS OF FUNCTIONING	
COMMUNICATION	
Healthy Families	› There are clear, understandable messages between family members, and each member is encouraged to express individual feelings and thoughts.
Dysfunctional Families	› One or more members use unhealthy patterns, such as:
	» Blaming – Members blame others to shift focus away from their own inadequacies.
	» Manipulating – Members use dishonesty to support their own agendas.
	» Placating – One member takes responsibility for problems to keep peace at all costs.
	» Distracting – A member inserts irrelevant information during attempts at problem solving.
MANAGEMENT	
Healthy Families	› Adults of a family agree on important issues, such as rule-making, finances, and plans for the future.
Dysfunctional Families	› Management can be chaotic, with a child making management decisions at times.
BOUNDARIES	
Healthy Families	› Boundaries are distinguishable between family roles. Clear boundaries define roles of each member and are understood by all. Each family member is able to function appropriately.
Dysfunctional Families	› Enmeshed boundaries – Thoughts, roles, and feelings blend so much that individual roles are unclear.
	› Rigid boundaries – Rules and roles are completely inflexible. These families tend to have members that isolate themselves.
SOCIALIZATION	
Healthy Families	› All members interact, plan, and adopt healthy ways of coping. Children learn to function as family members, as well as members of society. Members are able to change as the family grows and matures.
Dysfunctional Families	› Children do not learn healthy socialization skills within the family and have difficulty adapting to socialization roles of society.
EMOTIONAL/SUPPORTIVE	
Healthy Families	› Emotional needs of family members are met most of the time, and members have concerns about each other. Conflict and anger do not dominate.
Dysfunctional Families	› Negative emotions predominate most of time. Members are isolated, afraid, and do not show concern for each other.

- Other concepts related to family dysfunction
  - ○ Scapegoating – A member of the family who has little power is blamed for problems within the family. For example, one child who has not completed his chores might be blamed for the entire family not being able to go on an outing.
  - ○ Triangulation – A third party is drawn into the relationship with two members whose relationship is unstable. For example, one parent can develop an alliance with a child, leaving the other parent relatively uninvolved with both.
  - ○ Multigenerational issues – These are emotional issues or themes within a family that continue for at least three generations, such as a pattern of substance use or addictive behavior when the family is under stress, dysfunctional grief patterns, triangulation patterns, and divorce.

Family Therapy

- A family is defined as a group with reciprocal relationships in which members are committed to each other. Examples of a family vary widely and are often nontraditional, such as a family made up of a child living with her grown brother and his wife. Areas of functioning for families include management, boundaries, communication, emotional support, and socialization. Dysfunction can occur in any one or more areas.
- In family therapy, the focus is on the family as a system, rather than on each person as an individual.
- Nurses use focused interviews and use of various family assessment tools to collect data.

- Nurses work with families to reinforce teaching. For example, a nurse might provide reinforcement to a family regarding medication administration, or ways to help a family member manage his mental health disorder.
- Nurses also work to identify family resources, to improve communication, and to strengthen the family's ability to cope with the illness of one member.

FOCUS AND GOALS FOR INDIVIDUAL, FAMILY, AND GROUP THERAPIES	
FOCUS	GOALS
Individual	
› Client needs and problems › The therapeutic relationship	› Make more positive individual decisions. › Make productive life decisions. › Develop a strong sense of self.
Family	
› Family needs and problems within family dynamics › Improving family functioning	› Learn effective ways for dealing with mental illness within the family. › Improve understanding among family members. › Maximize positive interaction among family members.
Group	
› Helping individuals develop more functional and satisfying relations within a group setting	› Goals vary depending on type of group, but clients generally: » Discover that members share some common feelings, experiences, and thoughts. » Experience positive behavior changes as a result of group interaction and feedback.

APPLICATION EXERCISES

1. A nurse wants to use democratic leadership with a group whose purpose is to learn appropriate conflict-resolution techniques. The nurse is correct in implementing this form of group leadership when demonstrating which of the following actions?

    A. Observes group techniques without interfering with the group process

    B. Discusses a technique and then directs members to practice the technique

    C. Asks for group suggestions of techniques and then supports discussion

    D. Suggests techniques and asks group members to reflect on their use

2. A nurse is participating in group therapy for clients dealing with bereavement. Which of the following should the nurse include in the initial phase? (Select all that apply.)

_____ A. Encourage the group to work toward goals.

_____ B. Define the purpose of the group.

_____ C. Discuss termination of the group.

_____ D. Identify informal roles of members within the group.

_____ E. Establish an expectation of confidentiality within the group.

3. A nurse working on an acute mental health unit forms a group to focus on self-management of medications. At each of the meetings, two of the members use the opportunity to discuss their common interest in gambling on sports. This is an example of which of the following?

    A. Triangulation

    B. Group process

    C. Subgroup

    D. Hidden agenda

4. A nurse is participating in a family therapy session. The adolescent son tells the nurse that he plans ways to make his sister look bad so his parents will think he's the better sibling, which he believes will give him more privileges. The nurse should identify this dysfunctional behavior as which of the following?

    A. Placation

    B. Manipulation

    C. Blaming

    D. Distraction

5. A nurse is working with an established group and identifies various member roles. Which of the following should the nurse identify as an individual role?

    A. A member who praises input from other members

    B. A member who follows the direction of other members

    C. A member who brags about accomplishments

    D. A member who evaluates the group's performance toward a standard

6. A nurse is assisting with creating a plan of care for a family that is to begin therapy to improve the emotional and supportive aspect of the family unit. Use the ATI Active Learning Template: Basic Concept to complete this item to include the following sections:

    A. Related Content: Identify the definition of a family.

    B. Underlying Principles: Discuss the focus of family therapy.

    C. Nursing Interventions: Identify at least two interventions to assist the family during therapy.

APPLICATION EXERCISES KEY

1. A. INCORRECT: Laissez-faire leadership allows the group process to progress without any attempt by the leader to control the direction of the group.

    B. INCORRECT: Autocratic leadership controls the direction of the group.

    C. **CORRECT:** Democratic leadership supports group interaction and decision-making to solve problems.

    D. INCORRECT: Autocratic leadership controls the direction of the group.

    Ⓝ NCLEX® Connection: Psychosocial Integrity, Behavioral Management

2. A. INCORRECT: During the working phase, the group works toward goals.

    B. **CORRECT:** During the initial phase, the nurse should identify the purpose of the group.

    C. **CORRECT:** During the initial phase, the nurse should discuss termination of the group.

    D. INCORRECT: During the working phase, the nurse should identify informal roles that other members in the group often assume.

    E. **CORRECT:** During the initial phase, the nurse should set the tone of the group, including an expectation of confidentiality.

    Ⓝ NCLEX® Connection: Psychosocial Integrity, Behavioral Management

3. A. INCORRECT: Triangulation is when a third party is drawn into a relationship with two members whose relationship is unstable.

    B. INCORRECT: Group process is the verbal and nonverbal communication that occurs within the group during group sessions.

    C. INCORRECT: A subgroup is a small number of people within a larger group who function separately from that group.

    D. **CORRECT:** A hidden agenda is when some group members have a different goal than the stated group goals. The hidden agenda is often disruptive to the effective functioning of the group.

    Ⓝ NCLEX® Connection: Psychosocial Integrity, Behavioral Management

4. A. INCORRECT: Placation is the dysfunctional behavior of taking responsibility for problems to keep peace among family members.

    B. **CORRECT:** Manipulation is the dysfunctional behavior of using dishonesty to support an individual agenda.

    C. INCORRECT: Blaming is the dysfunctional behavior of blaming others to shift focus away from the individual's own inadequacies.

    D. INCORRECT: Distraction is the dysfunctional behavior of inserting irrelevant information during attempts at problem solving.

    (N) NCLEX® Connection: Psychosocial Integrity, Mental Health Concepts

5. A. INCORRECT: An individual who praises the input of others is acting in a maintenance role.

    B. INCORRECT: An individual who is a follower is acting in a maintenance role.

    C. **CORRECT:** An individual who brags about accomplishments is acting in an individual role that does not promote the progression of the group toward meeting goals.

    D. INCORRECT: An individual who evaluates the group's performance is acting in a task role.

    (N) NCLEX® Connection: Psychosocial Integrity, Behavioral Management

6. *Using the ATI Active Learning Template: Basic Concept*

    A. Related Content
    * A family is defined as a group with reciprocal relationships in which members are committed to each other.

    B. Underlying Principles
    * Family needs and problems within family dynamics
    * Improve family functioning

    C. Nursing Interventions
    * Encourage the family to use effective ways to deal with emotional needs of family members.
    * Assist the family to improve understanding among family members.
    * Promote positive interaction among family members.
    * Identify common feelings, experiences, and thoughts among family members.

    (N) NCLEX® Connection: Psychosocial Integrity, Support Systems

chapter 9

Overview

- Stress is the body's nonspecific response to any demand made upon it.
  - Stressors are physical or psychological factors that produce stress. Any stressor, whether it is perceived as "good" or "bad," produces a biological response in the body.
  - Individuals need the presence of some stressors to provide interest and purpose to life. However, too much stress or too many stressors can cause distress.
  - Anxiety and anger are damaging stressors that cause distress.
- General adaptation syndrome (GAS) is the body's response to an increased demand. The first stage is the initial adaptive response, also known as the "fight or flight" mechanism. If stress is prolonged, maladaptive responses can occur.
- Stress management is a person's ability to experience appropriate emotions and cope with stress.
  - The person who manages stress in a healthy manner is flexible and uses a variety of coping techniques or mechanisms.
  - Responses to stress and anxiety are affected by factors such as age, gender, culture, life experiences, and lifestyle.
  - The effects of stressors are cumulative. For example, the death of a family member can cause a high amount of stress. If the person experiencing that stress is also experiencing other stressful events at the same time, this could cause illness due to the cumulative effect of those stressors.
  - A person's ability to use successful stress management techniques can improve stress-related medical conditions and improve functioning.

Data Collection

- Protective factors increasing a person's resilience, or ability to resist the effects of stress, include the following.
  - Physical health
  - Strong sense of self
  - Religious or spiritual beliefs
  - Optimism
  - Hobbies and other outside interests
  - Satisfying interpersonal relationships
  - Strong social support systems
  - Humor

- Subjective and Objective Data

ACUTE STRESS (FIGHT OR FLIGHT)	PROLONGED STRESS (MALADAPTIVE RESPONSE)
› Apprehension	› Chronic anxiety or panic attacks
› Unhappiness or sorrow	› Depression, chronic pain, sleep disturbances
› Decreased appetite	› Weight gain or loss
› Increased respiratory rate, heart rate, cardiac output, blood pressure	› Increased risk for myocardial infarction, stroke
› Increased metabolism and glucose use	› Poor diabetes control, hypertension, fatigue, irritability, decreased ability to concentrate
› Depressed immune system	› Increased risk for infection

- Standardized Screening Tools
  - Life-changing events questionnaires, such as the Holmes and Rahe scale to measure Life Change Units, and Lazarus's Cognitive Appraisal

Patient-Centered Care

- Nursing Care
  - Most nursing care involves reinforcement of stress-reduction strategies to clients.
- Cognitive Techniques
  - Cognitive reframing
    - The client is helped to look at irrational cognitions (thoughts) in a more realistic light and to restructure those thoughts in a more positive way.
    - As an example, a client may think he is "a terrible father to my daughter." A health professional, using therapeutic communication techniques, could help the person reframe that thought into a positive thought, such as, "I've made some bad mistakes as a parent, but I've learned from them and have improved my parenting skills."
- Behavioral Techniques
  - Relaxation techniques
    - Meditation includes formal meditation techniques, as well as prayer for those who believe in a higher power.
    - Guided imagery – The client is guided through a series of images to promote relaxation. Images vary depending on the individual. For example, one client might imagine walking on a beach, while another client might imagine himself in a position of success.
    - Breathing exercises are used to decrease rapid breathing and promote relaxation.
    - Progressive muscle relaxation (PMR) – A person trained in this method can help a client attain complete relaxation within a few minutes.
    - Physical exercise (yoga, walking, biking) causes release of endorphins that lower anxiety, promote relaxation, and have antidepressant effects.
    - Use nursing judgement to determine the appropriateness of relaxation techniques for clients who are experiencing acute manifestations of a psychotic disorder.

- Journal writing
  - Journaling has been shown to allow for a therapeutic release of stress.
  - This activity can help the client identify stressors and make specific plans to decrease stressors.
- Priority restructuring
  - The client learns to prioritize differently to reduce the number of stressors affecting her.
  - For example, a person who is under stress due to feeling overworked might delegate some tasks to others rather than doing them all herself.
- Biofeedback
  - A nurse or other health professional trained in this method uses a sensitive mechanical device to assist the client to gain voluntary control of such autonomic functions as heart rate and blood pressure.
- Mindfulness
  - The client is encouraged to be mindful of his surroundings using all of his senses, such as the relaxing warmth of sunlight or the sound of a breeze blowing through the trees.
  - The client learns to restructure negative thoughts and interpretations into positive ones. For example, instead of saying, "It's so frustrating that the elevator isn't working," the client restructures the thought into, "Using the stairs is a great opportunity to burn off some extra calories."
- Assertiveness training
  - The client learns to communicate in a more assertive manner in order to decrease psychological stressors.
  - For example, one technique teaches the client to assert her feelings by describing a situation or behavior that causes stress, stating her feelings about the behavior or situation, and then making a change. The client states, "When you keep telling me what to do, I feel angry and frustrated. I need to try making some of my own decisions."
- Other individual stress-reduction techniques
  - The nurse should assist each client in identifying individual strategies that improve her ability to cope with stress.
    - Individual hobbies, such as fishing or scrapbooking
    - Music therapy
    - Pet therapy

APPLICATION EXERCISES

1. A nurse is preparing to attend an educational seminar on stress. Which of the following should be expected to be included in the discussion?

    A. Excessive stressors cause the client to experience distress.

    B. The body's initial adaptive response to stress is denial.

    C. The absence of stressors results in homeostasis.

    D. Negative, rather than positive, stressors produce a biological response.

2. A nurse is discussing acute vs. prolonged stress with a client. Which of the following should the nurse identify as an acute stress response? (Select all that apply.)

    _____ A. Decreased appetite

    _____ B. Depressed immune system

    _____ C. Increased blood pressure

    _____ D. Panic attacks

    _____ E. Unhappiness

3. A nurse is reinforcing teaching to a client about stress-reduction techniques. Which of the following client statements indicates understanding of the teaching?

    A. "Cognitive reframing will help me change my irrational thoughts to something positive."

    B. "Progressive muscle relaxation uses a mechanical device to help me gain control over my pulse rate."

    C. "Biofeedback causes my body to release endorphins so that I feel less stress and anxiety."

    D. "Mindfulness allows me to prioritize the stressors that I have in my life so that I have less anxiety."

4. A client says she is experiencing increased stress because her significant other is "pressuring me and my kids to go live with him. I love him, but I'm not ready to do that." She also states that her significant other "keeps nagging at my oldest son, which makes me mad, since he's my son, not his." Which of the following should the nurse recommend to promote a change in the client's situation?

    A. Learn to practice mindfulness.

    B. Use assertiveness techniques.

    C. Exercise regularly.

    D. Rely on the support of a close friend.

5. A nurse is caring for a client who states, "I'm so stressed at work because of my coworker. He expects me to finish his work because he's too lazy!" When discussing appropriate communication, which of the following statements by the client to his coworker indicates client understanding?

    A. "You really should complete your own work. I don't think it's right to expect me to complete your responsibilities."

    B. "Why do you expect me to finish your work? You must realize that I have my own responsibilities."

    C. "It is not fair to expect me to complete your work. If you continue, then I will report your behavior to our supervisor."

    D. "When I have to pick up extra work, I feel very overwhelmed. I need to focus on my own responsibilities."

6. A nurse is assisting with leading a peer group discussion about the general adaptation syndrome (GAS). Use the ATI Active Learning Template: Basic Concept and the Fundamentals Review Module to complete this item to include the following sections:

    A. Related Content: Define the GAS.

    B. Underlying Principles: Discuss the three stages of the GAS.

APPLICATION EXERCISES KEY

1. A. **CORRECT:** Distress is the result of excessive or damaging stressors, such as anxiety or anger.

    B. INCORRECT: Denial is part of the grief process. The body's initial adaptive response to stress is known as the fight-or-flight mechanism.

    C. INCORRECT: Individuals need the presence of some stressors to provide interest and purpose to life.

    D. INCORRECT: Both positive and negative stressors produce a biological response in the body.

    Ⓝ NCLEX® Connection: Psychosocial Integrity, Stress Management

2. A. **CORRECT:** Decreased appetite is an indicator of acute stress.

    B. **CORRECT:** A depressed immune system is an indicator of acute stress.

    C. **CORRECT:** Increased blood pressure is an indicator of acute stress.

    D. INCORRECT: Panic attacks indicate a prolonged or maladaptive stress response.

    E. **CORRECT:** Unhappiness is an indicator of acute stress.

    Ⓝ NCLEX® Connection: Psychosocial Integrity, Stress Management

3. A. **CORRECT:** Cognitive reframing helps the client look at irrational cognitions (thoughts) in a more realistic light and to restructure those thoughts in a more positive way.

    B. INCORRECT: Biofeedback, rather than progressive muscle training, uses a mechanical device to promote voluntary control over autonomic functions.

    C. INCORRECT: Physical exercise, rather than biofeedback, causes a release of endorphins that lower anxiety and reduce stress.

    D. INCORRECT: Priority restructuring, rather than mindfulness, teaches the client to prioritize differently to reduce the number of stressors.

    Ⓝ NCLEX® Connection: Psychosocial Integrity, Stress Management

4. A. INCORRECT: Mindfulness is appropriate to decrease the client's stress. However, it does not change the client's situation.

    B. **CORRECT:** Assertive communication allows the client to assert her feelings and then make a change in the situation.

    C. INCORRECT: Regular exercise is appropriate to decrease the client's stress. However, it does not change the client's situation.

    D. INCORRECT: Social support is appropriate to decrease the client's stress. However, it does not change the client's situation.

    Ⓝ NCLEX® Connection: Psychosocial Integrity, Stress Management

5. A. INCORRECT: This statement is an example of disapproving/disagreeing, which can prompt a defensive reaction and is therefore nontherapeutic.

    B. INCORRECT: This statement uses a "why" question, which implies criticism and can prompt a defensive reaction and is therefore nontherapeutic.

    C. INCORRECT: This statement is aggressive and threatening, which can prompt a defensive reaction and is therefore nontherapeutic.

    D. **CORRECT:** This response demonstrates assertive communication, which allows the client to state her feelings about the behavior and then promote a change.

    Ⓝ NCLEX® Connection: Psychosocial Integrity, Stress Management

6. *Using ATI Active Learning Template: Basic Concept*

    A. Related Content
    - The GAS is the body's response to an increased demand created by stressors.

    B. Underlying Principles
    - Stage 1 – Alarm Reaction: The alarm reaction is the body's initial adaptive response to a stressor. Also known as the fight-or-flight mechanism, body functions are heightened to respond to stressors. Indicators of the alarm reaction include elevated blood pressure and heart rate, heightened mental alertness, and increased secretion of epinephrine and norepinephrine.
    - Stage 2 – Resistance Stage: During the resistance stage, body functions normalize while responding to the stressor. The body attempts to cope with the stressor.
    - Stage 3 – Exhaustion Stage: If the client reaches the exhaustion stage, body functions are no longer able to maintain an adaptive response to the stressor.

    Ⓝ NCLEX® Connection: Psychosocial Integrity, Stress Management

chapter 10

Overview

- Brain stimulation therapies offer a nonpharmacological treatment for mental health disorders.
- Brain stimulation therapies include the following.
  - Electroconvulsive therapy (ECT)
    - ECT uses electrical current to induce brief seizure activity while the client is anesthetized.
    - The exact mechanism of ECT is still unknown. One theory suggests that the seizure activity produced by ECT can enhance the effects of neurotransmitters (serotonin, dopamine, and norepinephrine) in the brain.
  - Transcranial magnetic stimulation (TMS)
  - Vagus nerve stimulation (VNS)

ELECTROCONVULSIVE THERAPY (ECT)

Indications

- Major Depressive Disorder
  - Clients whose manifestations are not responsive to pharmacologic treatment
  - Clients for whom the risks of other treatments outweigh the risks of ECT, such as a client who is in her first trimester of pregnancy
  - Clients who are actively suicidal or homicidal and for whom there is a need for rapid therapeutic response
  - Clients who are experiencing psychotic manifestations
- Schizophrenia spectrum disorders that are less responsive to neuroleptic medications, such as schizoaffective disorder
- Acute Manic Episodes
  - ECT is used for clients who have bipolar disorder with rapid cycling (four or more episodes of acute mania within 1 year) and very destructive behavior. Both of these features tend to respond poorly to lithium therapy. These clients receive ECT and then a regimen of lithium therapy.

Contraindications

- There are no absolute contraindications for this therapy if it is deemed necessary to save a client's life. However, the nurse should be aware that some clients can have medical conditions that place them at higher risk if ECT is used. These conditions include the following.
  - Recent myocardial infarction
  - History of cerebrovascular accident
  - Cerebrovascular malformation
  - Intracranial mass lesion
  - Increased intracranial pressure
- Mental health conditions for which ECT has not been found useful include the following.
  - Substance use disorders
  - Personality disorders
  - Dysthymic disorder

Nursing Actions

- Preparation of the Client
  - The typical course of ECT treatment is three times a week for a total of six to 12 treatments.
  - The provider obtains informed consent.
    - If ECT is involuntary, consent can be obtained from next of kin or a court order.
  - Medication management

    - Any medications that affect the client's seizure threshold must be decreased or discontinued several days before the ECT procedure.
    - MAOIs and lithium should be discontinued 2 weeks before the ECT procedure.
  - Severe hypertension should be controlled because a short period of hypertension occurs immediately after the ECT procedure.
  - Any cardiac conditions, such as dysrhythmias, should be monitored and treated before the procedure.
  - The nurse monitors vital signs and mental status before and after the ECT procedure.

 M View Image: Electroconvulsive Therapy (ECT)

  - The nurse reinforces teaching as necessary based on the client's and family's understanding and knowledge of the procedure.
  - Thirty minutes prior to the beginning of the procedure, an IM injection of atropine sulfate or glycopyrrolate (Robinul) is given to decrease secretions and counteract any vagal stimulation.
  - An IV line is monitored and maintained until full recovery.

- Ongoing Care

    ○ ECT is administered early in the morning after the client has fasted for a prescribed period of time.

    ○ A bite guard should be used to prevent trauma to the oral cavity.

    ○ Electrodes are applied to the scalp, either unilaterally or bilaterally for encephalogram (EEG) monitoring.

    ○ The client is mechanically ventilated during the procedure and receives 100% oxygen.

    ○ Ongoing cardiac monitoring is provided, including blood pressure, electrocardiogram (ECG), and oxygen saturation.

    ○ An anesthesia provider administers a short-acting anesthetic, such as methohexital (Brevital), via IV bolus.

    ○ A muscle relaxant, such as succinylcholine (Anectine), is then administered.

    ○ A cuff is placed on one leg or arm to block the muscle relaxant so that seizure activity can be monitored in the limb distal to the cuff.

    ○ The electrical stimulus is typically applied for 0.2 to 0.8 seconds. Seizure activity is monitored, and the duration of the seizure (usually 25 to 60 seconds) is documented.

    ○ After seizure activity has ceased, the anesthetic is discontinued.

    ○ The client is extubated and assisted to breathe voluntarily.

- Postprocedure Care

    ○ When stable, the client is transferred to a recovery area where level of consciousness, cardiac status, vital signs, and oxygen saturation continue to be monitored.

    ○ The client is positioned on his side to facilitate drainage and prevent aspiration.

    ○ The client is monitored for ability to swallow and return of the gag reflex.

    ○ The client is usually awake and ready for transfer back to the mental health unit or other facility within 30 to 60 min after the procedure.

Complications

- Memory Loss and Confusion

    ○ Short-term memory loss, confusion, and disorientation can occur immediately following the procedure. Memory loss can persist for several weeks. Whether ECT causes permanent memory loss is controversial.

    ○ Nursing actions

        ▪ Provide frequent orientation.

        ▪ Provide a safe environment to prevent injury.

        ▪ Assist with personal hygiene as needed.

- Reactions to Anesthesia
  - Nursing actions
    - Provide continuous monitoring during the procedure and in the immediate recovery phase.
- ECG Changes
  - The client's baseline heart rate is expected to increase by 25% during the procedure and early recovery.
  - Blood pressure can fall initially and then rise during the procedure. The elevated blood pressure should resolve shortly after the procedure.
  - Nursing actions
    - Monitor vital signs regularly per protocol.
    - Orient the client as necessary.
- Headache, muscle soreness, and nausea can occur during and following the immediate recovery period
  - Nursing actions
    - Observe the client to determine the degree of discomfort.
    - Administer antiemetic and analgesic medications as needed.
- Relapse of depression
  - Advise the client that ECT is not a permanent cure.
  - Weekly or monthly maintenance ECT can decrease the incidence of relapse.

TRANSCRANIAL MAGNETIC STIMULATION (TMS)

- TMS is a noninvasive therapy that uses magnetic pulsations to stimulate specific areas of the brain.

Indications

- Major depressive disorder
  - Clients who are not responsive to pharmacologic treatment

Nursing Actions

- Reinforce teaching to the client about TMS.
  - TMS commonly is prescribed daily for a period of 4 to 6 weeks.
  - TMS can be performed as an outpatient procedure.
  - The TMS procedure lasts 30 to 40 min.
  - A noninvasive electromagnet is placed on the client's scalp, allowing the magnetic pulsations to pass through.
  - The client is alert during the procedure.

Complications

- Common adverse effects include mild discomfort or a tingling sensation at the site of the electromagnet.
- Monitor the client for lightheadedness after the procedure.
- Seizures are a rare but potential complication.
- TMS is not associated with systemic adverse effects or neurologic deficits.

VAGUS NERVE STIMULATION (VNS)

- VNS provides electrical stimulation through the vagus nerve to the brain through a device that is surgically implanted under the skin on the client's chest.
- VNS is believed to result in an increased level of neurotransmitters.

Indications

- Depression that is resistant to pharmacological treatment and/or ECT.
- Current research studies are determining the effectiveness for VNS in clients who have anxiety disorders.

Nursing Actions

- Reinforce teaching to the client about VNS.
  - ○ VNS commonly is performed as an outpatient surgical procedure.
  - ○ The VNS device delivers around-the-clock programmed pulsations.
  - ○ The client can turn off the VNS device at any time by placing a special external magnet over the site of the implant.
- Assist the provider in obtaining informed consent.

Complications

- Voice changes due to the proximity of the implanted lead on the vagus nerve to the larynx and pharynx.
- Other potential adverse effects include hoarseness, throat or neck pain, dysphagia. These commonly improve with time.
- Dyspnea, especially with physical exertion, is possible. Therefore, the client might want to turn off the VNS during exercise.

APPLICATION EXERCISES

1. A nurse is reinforcing teaching with a client who is scheduled to receive electroconvulsive therapy (ECT) for the treatment of major depressive disorder. Which of the following client statements indicates understanding of the teaching?

    A. "It is common to treat depression with ECT before trying medications."

    B. "I can have my depression cured if I receive a series of ECT treatments."

    C. "I will have seizures lasting 1½ to 2 minutes during ECT."

    D. "I will receive a muscle relaxant to protect me from injury during ECT."

2. A nurse is discussing transcranial magnetic stimulation (TMS) with a newly licensed nurse. Which of the following statements by the newly licensed nurse indicates a need for further teaching?

    A. "TMS is indicated for clients whose depression is not relieved by medication."

    B. "I will provide postanesthesia care following TMS."

    C. "TMS is usually performed as an outpatient procedure."

    D. "I will schedule the client for daily TMS treatments for the first several weeks."

3. A nurse is monitoring a client immediately following an electroconvulsive therapy (ECT) procedure. Which of the following are expected findings? (Select all that apply.)

    _____ A. Hypotension

    _____ B. Paralytic ileus

    _____ C. Memory loss

    _____ D. Nausea

    _____ E. Tachycardia

4. A nurse is leading a peer group discussion about the indications for electroconvulsive therapy (ECT). Which of the following is appropriate to include in the discussion?

    A. Borderline personality disorder

    B. Acute withdrawal related to a substance use disorder

    C. Bipolar disorder with rapid cycling

    D. Dysthymic disorder

5. A nurse is assisting with the planning of care for a client following surgical implantation of a vagus nerve stimulation (VNS) device. The nurse should monitor for which of the following adverse effects? (Select all that apply.)

_____ A. Voice changes

_____ B. Seizure activity

_____ C. Disorientation

_____ D. Dysphagia

_____ E. Neck pain

6. A nurse is preparing to assist in providing electroconvulsive therapy (ECT) treatment for a client. Use the ATI Active Learning Template: Therapeutic Procedure to complete this item to include the following sections:

A. Description of Procedure

B. Nursing Actions: Identify two preprocedure medication management actions.

C. Nursing Actions: Identify at least three intraprocedure actions.

APPLICATION EXERCISES KEY

1. A. INCORRECT: ECT is indicated for clients who have major depressive disorder and who are not responsive to pharmacologic treatment.

    B. INCORRECT: ECT does not cure depression. However, it can reduce the incidence and severity of relapse.

    C. INCORRECT: Induced seizures during ECT typically last only 25 to 60 seconds.

    D. **CORRECT:** A muscle relaxant, such as succinylcholine (Anectine), is administered to reduce the risk for injury during induced seizure activity.

    Ⓝ NCLEX® Connection: Reduction of Risk Potential, Potential for Complications of Diagnostic Tests/ Treatments/Procedures

2. A. INCORRECT: This statement does not require further teaching. TMS is indicated for the treatment of major depressive disorder that is not responsive to pharmacologic treatment.

    B. **CORRECT:** This statement requires further teaching. Postanesthesia care is not necessary after TMS because the client does not receive anesthesia and is alert during the procedure.

    C. INCORRECT: This statement does not require further teaching. TMS is noninvasive and can be performed as an outpatient procedure.

    D. INCORRECT: This statement does not require further teaching. TMS is commonly prescribed daily for a period of 4 to 6 weeks.

    Ⓝ NCLEX® Connection: Reduction of Risk Potential, Potential for Complications of Diagnostic Tests/ Treatments/Procedures

3. A. INCORRECT: Immediately following ECT, the client's blood pressure is expected to be elevated.

    B. INCORRECT: Paralytic ileus is not an expected finding of ECT.

    C. **CORRECT:** Transient short-term memory loss is an expected finding immediately following ECT.

    D. **CORRECT:** Nausea is an expected finding immediately following ECT.

    E. **CORRECT:** Tachycardia is an expected finding immediately following ECT.

    Ⓝ NCLEX® Connection: Reduction of Risk Potential, Potential for Complications of Diagnostic Tests/ Treatments/Procedures

4. A. INCORRECT: ECT has not been found to be effective for the treatment of personality disorders.

    B. INCORRECT: ECT has not been found to be effective for the treatment of substance use disorders.

    C. **CORRECT:** ECT is indicated for the treatment of bipolar disorder with rapid cycling.

    D. INCORRECT: ECT has not been found effective for the treatment of dysthymic disorder.

    Ⓝ NCLEX® Connection: Reduction of Risk Potential, Potential for Complications of Diagnostic Tests/ Treatments/Procedures

5.   A. **CORRECT:** Voice changes are a common adverse effect of VNS due to the proximity of the implanted lead on the vagus nerve to the larynx and pharynx.

   B. INCORRECT: Seizure activity is associated with ECT rather than VNS.

   C. INCORRECT: Disorientation is associated with ECT and TMS rather than VNS.

   D. **CORRECT:** Dysphagia is a potential adverse effect of VNS. However, this usually subsides with time.

   E. **CORRECT:** Neck pain is a potential adverse effect of VNS. However, this usually subsides with time.

   (N) NCLEX® Connection: Reduction of Risk Potential, Potential for Complications of Diagnostic Tests/Treatments/Procedures

6.   *Using ATI Active Learning Template: Therapeutic Procedure*

   A. Description of Procedure
   - ECT is a nonpharmacologic brain stimulation therapy for the treatment of mental health disorders, especially major depressive disorder. ECT induces seizure activity, which is thought to enhance the effects of neurotransmitters in the brain.

   B. Nursing Actions: Preprocedure medication management actions
   - Several days before ECT, discontinue any medications affecting the client's seizure threshold.
   - Discontinue MAOIs 2 weeks prior to ECT.
   - Discontinue lithium 2 weeks prior to ECT.
   - Administer atropine sulfate or glycopyrrolate (Robinul) IM 30 min prior to ECT.
   - Monitor IV access prior to ECT.

   C. Nursing Actions: Intraprocedure actions
   - Place a bite guard to prevent trauma to the oral cavity.
   - Apply electrodes to the scalp for encephalogram (EEG) monitoring.
   - Apply cardiac electrodes for ECT monitoring.
   - Place a cuff on one leg or arm to monitor for distal seizure activity.
   - Monitor and document seizure activity.
   - Monitor vital signs.
   - Position the client on his side after extubation to facilitate drainage and prevent aspiration.

   (N) NCLEX® Connection: Reduction of Risk Potential, Potential for Complications of Diagnostic Tests/Treatments/Procedures

UNIT 3   Psychobiologic Disorders

CHAPTERS

› Anxiety Disorders
› Depressive Disorders
› Bipolar Disorders
› Psychotic Disorders
› Personality Disorders
› Cognitive Disorders
› Substance Use and Addictive Disorders
› Eating Disorders

NCLEX® CONNECTIONS

When reviewing the chapters in this unit, keep in mind the relevant sections of the NCLEX® outline, in particular:

Client Needs: Psychosocial Integrity

› Relevant topics/tasks include:
  » Crisis Intervention
    › Identify the client in crisis.
  » Behavioral Management
    › Assist the client in using behavioral strategies to decrease anxiety.
  » Mental Health Concepts
    › Identify the client's symptoms of acute or chronic mental illness.
    › Assist in the care of the cognitively impaired client.
  » Therapeutic Communication
    › Encourage the client's appropriate use of verbal and non-verbal communication.
  » Therapeutic Environment
    › Contribute to maintaining a safe and supportive environment for the client.

Client Needs: Pharmacological Therapies

› Relevant topics/tasks include:
  » Adverse Effects/Contraindications/Interactions
    › Monitor the client for actual and potential adverse effects of medications.
  » Expected Actions/Outcomes
    › Reinforce education to the client regarding medications.

chapter 11

Overview

- Normal anxiety is a healthy response to stress that is essential for survival. Elevated or persistent anxiety can result in anxiety disorders causing behavior changes and impairment in functioning. Anxiety disorders tend to be persistent and are often disabling.

- Anxiety levels can be mild (restlessness, increased motivation, irritability), moderate (agitation, muscle tightness), severe (inability to function, ritualistic behavior, unresponsive), or panic (distorted perception, loss of rational thought, immobility).

- The various anxiety disorders recognized and defined by the DSM-5 include the following.

    ○ Separation anxiety disorder – The client experiences excessive fear or anxiety when separated from an individual to which to client is emotionally attached.

    ○ Panic disorder – The client experiences recurrent panic attacks.

    ○ Phobias – The client fears a specific object or situation to an unreasonable level.

    ○ Generalized anxiety disorder (GAD) – The client exhibits uncontrollable, excessive worry for more than 3 months.

- Other disorders not specifically identified by the DSM-5 as anxiety disorders but have similar effects include the following.

    ○ Obsessive-compulsive and related disorders

        ▪ Obsessive compulsive disorder (OCD) – The client has intrusive thoughts of unrealistic obsessions and tries to control these thoughts with compulsive behaviors (for example, repetitive cleaning of a particular object or washing of hands).

        ▪ Hoarding disorder – The client has difficulty parting with possessions, resulting in extreme stress and functional impairments.

    ○ Trauma- and stressor-related disorders

        ▪ Acute stress disorder – Exposure to a traumatic event causes numbing, detachment, and amnesia about the event for at least 3 days but for not more than 1 month following the event.

        ▪ Posttraumatic stress disorder (PTSD) – Exposure to a traumatic event causes intense fear, horror, flashbacks, feelings of detachment and foreboding, restricted affect, and impairment for longer than 1 month after the event. Manifestations can last for years.

Data Collection

- Risk Factors

  - Anxiety disorders are much more likely to occur in women. OCD has equal prevalence in men and women.

  - Anxiety, obsessive-compulsive, and even trauma- and stressor-related disorders have a genetic and neurobiological link.

  - Exposure to a traumatic event or experience, such as military combat or threat of death of a loved one, can precipitate an anxiety, or trauma- and stressor-related disorder.

  - Anxiety can be due to an acute medical condition, such as hyperthyroidism or pulmonary embolism. It is important to monitor the manifestations of anxiety in an appropriate medical facility to rule out a physical cause.

  - Adverse effects of many medications can mimic anxiety disorders.

  - Substance-induced anxiety is related to current use of a chemical substance, or to withdrawal effects from a substance, such as alcohol.

- Subjective and Objective Data

  - Panic disorder

    - Panic attacks typically last 15 to 30 min.

    - Four or more of the following manifestations are present during a panic attack.

      - Palpitations

      - Shortness of breath

      - Choking or smothering sensation

      - Chest pain

      - Nausea

      - Feelings of depersonalization

      - Fear of dying or insanity

      - Chills or hot flashes

    - The client can experience behavior changes and/or persistent worries about when the next attack will occur.

  - Phobias

    - Social phobia – The client has a fear of embarrassment, is unable to perform in front of others, has a dread of social situations, believes that others are judging him negatively, and has impaired relationships.

    - Agoraphobia – The client avoids being outside and has an impaired ability to work or perform duties.

    - Specific phobias

      - The client has a fear of specific objects, such as spiders, snakes, strangers.

      - The client has a fear of specific experiences, such as flying, being in the dark, riding in an elevator, being in an enclosed space.

- Generalized anxiety disorder (GAD) – The client exhibits uncontrollable, excessive worry for more than 3 months.
  - GAD causes significant impairment in one or more areas of functioning, such as work-related duties.
  - Manifestations of GAD include the following.
    - Restlessness
    - Muscle tension
    - Avoidance of stressful activities or events
    - Increased time and effort required to prepare for stressful activities or events
    - Procrastination in decision-making
    - Seeks repeated reassurance
- Obsessive-compulsive and related disorders
  - OCD – Persistent thoughts or urges that the client attempts to suppress through compulsive or obsessive behaviors. Obsessions or compulsions are time-consuming and result in impaired social and occupational functioning.
  - Hoarding disorder – Client has obsessive desire to save items regardless of value. Experiences extreme stress with thoughts of discarding or getting rid of items. Client's hoarding behavior results in social and occupational impairment and often leads to an unsafe living environment.
- Trauma – and stressor-related disorders

ACUTE STRESS DISORDER	PTSD
Precipitating event	
› In both disorders, the client witnesses or experiences an actual event that threatens severe injury or death to the client or others. › The client responds with fear, helplessness, or horror to the event.	
Onset and duration	
› Manifestations often begin immediately following the traumatic event and persist for at least 3 days. Duration is 3 days to 1 month.	› Manifestations can occur any time following the traumatic event with potential delays of months or years. The duration of manifestations last more than 1 month.
Reexperience of the event	
› The client persistently reexperiences the event through: » Distress when reminded of the event » Dreams or images » Reliving through flashbacks	› The client persistently reexperiences the event through: » Recurrent, intrusive recollection of the event » Dreams or images » Reliving through flashbacks, illusions, or hallucinations
Manifestations	
› Dissociative manifestations, such as amnesia of the trauma event, absent emotional response, decreased awareness of surroundings, depersonalization › Indications of severe anxiety, such as irritability, sleep disturbance	› Indications of increased arousal, such as irritability, difficulty with concentration, sleep disturbance › Avoidance of stimuli associated with trauma, such as avoiding people, inability to show feelings

- Standardized Screening Tools
  - Hamilton Rating Scale for Anxiety
  - Modified Spielberger State Anxiety Scale
  - Yale-Brown Obsessive-Compulsive Scale
  - Hoarding Scale Self-Report
  - National Stressful Events Survey

Patient-Centered Care

- Nursing Care
  - Provide a structured interview to keep the client focused on the present.
  - Collect data and document comorbid condition of substance use disorder.
  - Provide safety and comfort to the client during the crisis period of these disorders, as clients in severe- to panic-level anxiety are unable to problem solve and focus.
  - Remain with the client during the worst of the anxiety to provide reassurance.
  - Collect data and document suicide risk.
  - Provide a safe environment for other clients and staff.
  - Provide milieu therapy that employs the following.
    - A structured environment for physical safety and predictability
    - Monitoring for, and protection from, self-harm or suicide
    - Daily activities that encourage the client to share and be cooperative
    - Use of therapeutic communication skills, such as open-ended questions, to help the client express feelings of anxiety, and to validate and acknowledge those feelings
    - Client participation in decision making regarding care
  - Use relaxation techniques with the client as needed for relief of pain, muscle tension, and feelings of anxiety.
  - Instill hope for positive outcomes (but avoid false reassurance).
  - Enhance client self-esteem by encouraging positive statements and discussing past achievements.
  - Assist the client to identify defense mechanisms that interfere with recovery.
  - Postpone health teaching until after acute anxiety subsides. Clients experiencing a panic attack or severe anxiety are unable to concentrate or learn.

  - Specific therapies include the following:
    - Cognitive behavioral therapy – The anxiety response can be decreased by changing cognitive distortions. This therapy uses cognitive reframing to help the client identify negative thoughts that produce anxiety, examine the cause, and develop supportive ideas that replace negative self-talk.
    - Behavioral therapies teach clients ways to decrease anxiety or avoidant behavior and allow an opportunity to practice techniques.
      - Relaxation training is used to control pain, tension, and anxiety. Refer to the chapter on *Stress Management*, which covers relaxation training techniques.
      - Modeling allows a client to see a demonstration of appropriate behavior in a stressful situation. The goal of therapy is that the client will imitate the behavior.

- □ Systematic desensitization begins with mastering of relaxation techniques. Then, a client is exposed to increasing levels of an anxiety-producing stimulus (either imagined or real) and uses relaxation to overcome the resulting anxiety. The goal of therapy is that the client is able to tolerate a greater and greater level of the stimulus until anxiety no longer interferes with functioning. This form of therapy is especially effective for clients who have phobias.

- □ Flooding involves exposing the client to a great deal of an undesirable stimulus in an attempt to turn off the anxiety response. This therapy is most useful for clients who have phobias.

- □ Response prevention focuses on preventing the client from performing a compulsive behavior with the intent that anxiety will diminish.

- □ Thought stopping teaches a client to say "stop" when negative thoughts or compulsive behaviors arise, and substitute a positive thought. The goal of therapy is that with time, the client uses the command silently.

  - ▪ Group and family therapy is beneficial, especially for clients who have trauma- and stressor-related disorders.

  - ▪ Eye movement desensitization and reprocessing (EMDR) is a therapy for clients who have PTSD. EMDR encourages eye focus on a separate stimuli while thinking of or talking about the traumatic event.

- Medications

  - ○ SSRI antidepressants, such as sertraline (Zoloft), are the first line of treatment for trauma- and stressor-related disorders. Clients who have anxiety disorders also can benefit from other types of antidepressants.

  - ○ Sedative hypnotic anxiolytics, such as diazepam (Valium), are indicated for short-term use.

  - ○ Nonbarbiturate anxiolytics, such as buspirone, are used to manage anxiety.

  - ○ Other medications that can be used to treat anxiety disorders include beta-blockers and antihistamines to decrease anxiety. Anticonvulsants are used as mood stabilizers for the client who is experiencing anxiety.

- Care After Discharge

  - ○ Reinforce Client Education

    - ▪ Reinforce client education regarding identification of manifestations of anxiety.

    - ▪ Tell the client to notify the provider of worsening effects and to not adjust medication dosages. Warn the client against stopping or increasing medication without consultation with the provider.

    - ▪ Assist the client to evaluate coping mechanisms that work and do not work for controlling the anxiety, and assist the client to learn new methods. Use of alternative stress relief and coping mechanisms can increase medication effectiveness and decrease the need for medication in most cases.

APPLICATION EXERCISES

1. A nurse is caring for a client who has acute stress disorder and is experiencing severe anxiety. Which of the following statements by the nurse is appropriate?

    A. "Tell me about how you are feeling right now."

    B. "You should focus on the positive things in your life to decrease your anxiety."

    C. "Why do you believe you are experiencing this anxiety?"

    D. "Let's discuss the medications your provider is prescribing to decrease your anxiety."

2. A nurse observes a client who has OCD repeatedly applying, removing, and then reapplying makeup. Repetitive behavior in a client who has OCD is due to which of the following?

    A. Narcissistic behavior

    B. Fear of rejection from staff

    C. Attempt to reduce anxiety

    D. Adverse effect of antidepressant medication

3. A nurse is caring for a client who is experiencing a panic attack. Which of the following is an appropriate nursing intervention?

    A. Discuss new relaxation techniques.

    B. Show the client how to change his behavior.

    C. Distract the client with a television show.

    D. Stay with the client, and remain quiet.

4. A nurse observes a client who is pacing and wringing his hands. The client states, "I don't know why, but I've worried every day for over a year that my son will die a horrible death." This finding is consistent with which of the following disorders?

    A. Generalized anxiety disorder

    B. Panic disorder

    C. Posttraumatic stress disorder

    D. Acute stress disorder

5. A nurse working on an acute mental health unit is caring for a client who has posttraumatic stress disorder (PTSD). Which of the following are expected findings? (Select all that apply.)

_____ A. Hallucinations

_____ B. Obsessive need to talk about the traumatic event

_____ C. Exaggerated displays of emotion

_____ D. Recurring nightmares

_____ E. Diminished reflexes

6. A nurse working in a mental health clinic is reinforcing teaching for a client who has a phobia of riding on an elevator about the use of systematic desensitization as a form of behavioral therapy. Use the ATI Active Learning Template: Therapeutic Procedure to complete this item to include the following sections:

A. Description of Procedure

B. Indications: Describe one.

APPLICATION EXERCISES KEY

1.   A. **CORRECT:** Asking an open-ended question is therapeutic and assists the client in identifying anxiety.

    B. INCORRECT: Offering advice is nontherapeutic and can hinder further communication.

    C. INCORRECT: Asking the client a "why" question is nontherapeutic and can promote a defensive client response.

    D. INCORRECT: Postpone health teaching until after acute anxiety subsides. Clients experiencing severe anxiety are unable to concentrate or learn.

    (N) NCLEX® Connection: Psychosocial Integrity, Therapeutic Communication

2.   A. INCORRECT: Clients who have OCD demonstrate repetitive behavior but not narcissism, which can be associated with personality disorders.

    B. INCORRECT: Clients who have OCD demonstrate repetitive behavior but not fear of rejection, which can be associated with social phobias.

    C. **CORRECT:** Clients who have OCD demonstrate repetitive behavior in an attempt to suppress persistent thoughts or urges.

    D. INCORRECT: Clients who have OCD can take an antidepressant to help control repetitive behavior.

    (N) NCLEX® Connection: Psychosocial Integrity, Behavioral Management

3.   A. INCORRECT: During a panic attack, the client is unable to concentrate on learning new information.

    B. INCORRECT: During a panic attack, the client is unable to concentrate on learning new information.

    C. INCORRECT: During a panic attack, the nurse should maintain a calm, quiet environment. Further stimuli can increase the client's level of anxiety.

    D. **CORRECT:** During a panic attack, the nurse should quietly remain with the client. This promotes safety and reassurance without additional stimuli.

    (N) NCLEX® Connection: Psychosocial Integrity, Behavioral Management

4. A. **CORRECT:** Generalized anxiety disorder is characterized by uncontrollable, excessive worry for more than 3 months.

    B. INCORRECT: Panic disorder is associated with recurrent panic attacks rather than chronic worrying.

    C. INCORRECT: PTSD is associated with a specific traumatic event.

    D. INCORRECT: Acute stress disorder is associated with a specific traumatic event.

    Ⓝ NCLEX® Connection: Psychosocial Integrity, Mental Health Concepts

5. A. **CORRECT:** Hallucinations associated with the traumatic event are an expected finding of PTSD.

    B. INCORRECT: Avoidance of stimuli associated with the traumatic event is an expected finding of PTSD.

    C. INCORRECT: The inability to show feelings or emotions is an expected finding of PTSD.

    D. **CORRECT:** Recurring nightmares associated with the traumatic event are an expected finding of PTSD.

    E. INCORRECT: Increased arousal, rather than diminished reflexes, is an expected finding of PTSD.

    Ⓝ NCLEX® Connection: Psychosocial Integrity, Mental Health Concepts

6. *Using the ATI Active Learning Template: Therapeutic Procedure*

    A. Description of Procedure
    - Systematic desensitization is a behavioral therapy that exposes clients to increasing levels of an anxiety-producing stimulus.

    B. Indication
    - Systematic desensitization is indicated for the treatment of phobias or other anxiety disorders associated with an anxiety-producing stimulus.

    Ⓝ NCLEX® Connection: Psychosocial Integrity, Behavioral Management

chapter 12

Overview

- Depression is a mood (affective) disorder that is a widespread issue, ranking high among causes of disability.
- Depression can be comorbid with the following.
  - Anxiety disorders
    - These disorders are comorbid in approximately 70% of clients who have a depressive disorder. This combination makes a client's prognosis poorer, with a higher risk for suicide and disability.
  - Psychotic disorders, such as schizophrenia
  - Substance use disorder
    - Clients often use substances in an attempt to relieve manifestations of depression and/or self-treat mental health disorders.
  - Eating disorders
  - Personality disorders
- A client who has depression has a potential risk for suicide, especially if he has a family or personal history of suicide attempts, comorbid anxiety disorder or panic attacks, comorbid substance use disorder or psychosis, poor self-esteem, a lack of social support, or a chronic medical condition.
- Depressive disorders recognized and defined by the DSM-5
  - Major depressive disorder (MDD) is a single episode or recurrent episodes of unipolar depression (not associated with mood swings from major depression to mania) resulting in a significant change in a client's normal functioning (social, occupational, self-care) accompanied by at least five of the following specific clinical findings, which must occur almost every day for a minimum of 2 weeks and last most of the day.
    - Depressed mood
    - Difficulty sleeping or excessive sleeping
    - Indecisiveness
    - Decreased ability to concentrate
    - Suicidal ideation
    - Increase or decrease in motor activity
    - Inability to feel pleasure
    - Increase or decrease in weight of more than 5% of total body weight over 1 month

○ MDD can be further diagnosed in the DSM-5 with a more specific classification.

- Psychotic features – the presence of auditory hallucinations (for example, voices telling the client she is sinful) or the presence of delusions (for example, client thinking that she has a fatal disease)

- Postpartum onset – a depressive episode that begins within 4 weeks of childbirth (known as postpartum depression) and can include delusions, which can put the newborn infant at high risk of being harmed by the mother

- Seasonal characteristics – seasonal affective disorder (SAD), which occurs during winter and can be treated with light therapy

○ Dysthymic disorder is a milder form of depression that usually has an early onset, such as in childhood or adolescence, and lasts at least 2 years in length for adults (1 year in length for children). Dysthymic disorder contains at least three clinical findings of depression, and can become major depressive disorder later in life.

○ Premenstrual dysphoric disorder (PMDD) is a depressive disorder associated with the luteal phase of the menstrual cycle. Primary manifestations include emotional lability and persistent or severe anger and irritability. Other manifestations include a lack of energy, overeating, and difficulty concentrating.

- Care of a client who has MDD will mirror the phase of the disease that the client is experiencing.

PHASE	CHARACTERISTICS	TREATMENT
Acute	› Severe clinical findings of depression	› Treatment is generally 6 to 12 weeks in duration. › There is a potential need for hospitalization. › Reduction of depressive manifestations is the goal of treatment. › Monitor for suicide risk, and implement safety precautions or one-to-one observation as needed.
Continuation	› Increased ability to function	› Treatment is generally 4 to 9 months in duration. › Relapse prevention through education, medication therapy, and psychotherapy is the goal of treatment.
Maintenance	› Remission of manifestations	› This phase can last for years. › Prevention of future depressive episodes is the goal of treatment.

Data Collection

- Risk Factors

○ Family history and a personal history of depression are the most significant risk factors.

○ Depressive disorders are twice as common in females between the ages of 15 and 40 than in males.

○ Depression is very common among clients older than age 65, but the disorder is more difficult to recognize in the older adult client and can go untreated. It is important to differentiate between early dementia and depression. Some clinical findings of depression that can look like dementia are memory loss, confusion, and behavioral problems, such as social isolation or agitation. Clients can seek health care for somatic problems that are manifestations of untreated depression.

- ○ Neurotransmitter deficiencies
  - ▪ Serotonin deficiency, which affects mood, sexual behavior, sleep cycles, hunger, and pain perception
  - ▪ Norepinephrine deficiency, which affects attention and behavior
- ○ Other risk factors
  - ▪ Stressful life events
  - ▪ Presence of a medical illness
  - ▪ Being a female in the postpartum period
  - ▪ Poor social support network
  - ▪ Comorbid substance use disorder
  - ▪ Being unmarried
- ○ Depressive disorders occur in all groups of people.
- ○ Depression can be the primary disorder, or it can be a response to another physical or mental health disorder.
- • Subjective Data
  - ○ Anergia (lack of energy)
  - ○ Anhedonia (lack of pleasure in normal activities)
  - ○ Anxiety
  - ○ Reports of sluggishness (most common), or feeling unable to relax and sit still
  - ○ Vegetative findings, which include a change in eating patterns (usually anorexia in MDD, increased intake in dysthymia and PMDD), change in bowel habits (usually constipation), sleep disturbances, and decreased interest in sexual activity
  - ○ Somatic reports, such as fatigue, gastrointestinal changes, pain
- • Objective Data
  - ○ Physical findings
    - ▪ Affect – The client most often looks sad with blunted affect.
    - ▪ The client exhibits poor grooming and lack of hygiene.
    - ▪ Psychomotor retardation (slowed physical movement, slumped posture) is more common, but psychomotor agitation (restlessness, pacing, finger tapping) also can occur.
    - ▪ The client becomes socially isolated, showing little or no effort to interact.
    - ▪ Slowed speech, decreased verbalization, delayed response – The client can seem too tired even to speak.

 View Video: Understanding Major Depression

- Standardized Screening Tools
  - ○ Hamilton Depression Scale
  - ○ Beck Depression Inventory

  - ○ Geriatric Depression Scale (short form)
  - ○ Zung Self-Rating Depression Scale
  - ○ Confidential screening tool at www.mentalhealthamerica.net/llw/depression_screen.cfm

Patient-Centered Care

- Nursing Care
  - ○ Milieu Therapy
    - ▪ Suicide risk – Check the client's risk for suicide, and implement appropriate safety precautions.
    - ▪ Self-care – Monitor the client's ability to perform activities of daily living, and encourage independence as much as possible.
    - ▪ Communication
      - ▫ Relate therapeutically to the client who is unable or unwilling to communicate.
        - ‣ Make time to be with the client, even if he does not speak.
        - ‣ Make observations rather than asking direct questions, which can cause anxiety in the client. For example, the nurse might say, "I noticed that you attended the unit group meeting today," rather than asking, "Did you enjoy the group meeting?" Give directions in simple, concrete sentences because a client who has depression can have difficulty focusing on and comprehending long sentences.
        - ‣ Give the client sufficient time to respond when holding a conversation due to a possible delayed response time.
    - ▪ Maintenance of a safe environment
    - ▪ Counseling, which can include individual counseling to assist with the following
      - ▫ Problem solving
      - ▫ Increasing coping abilities
      - ▫ Changing negative thinking to positive
      - ▫ Increasing self-esteem
      - ▫ Assertiveness training
      - ▫ Using available community resources

- Medications
  - Antidepressants
    - Reinforce client teaching for all antidepressants.

      - Do not discontinue medication suddenly.
      - Therapeutic effects are not immediate. It can take several weeks or more to reach full therapeutic benefits.
      - Avoid hazardous activities, such as driving or operating heavy equipment/machinery, due to the potential adverse effect of sedation.
      - Notify the provider of any thoughts of suicide.
      - Avoid alcohol while taking an antidepressant.

MEDICATION CLASSIFICATION/EXAMPLE	REINFORCE CLIENT TEACHING
› Selective serotonin reuptake inhibitors (SSRIs) » Citalopram (Celexa) » Fluoxetine (Prozac) » Sertraline (Zoloft)	› Adverse effects can include nausea, headache, and CNS stimulation (agitation, insomnia, anxiety). › Sexual dysfunction can occur. Notify provider if effects are intolerable. › Observe for manifestations of serotonin syndrome. If any occur, withhold the medication and notify the provider. › Avoid the concurrent use of St. John's wort, which can increase the risk of serotonin syndrome. › Follow a healthy diet because weight gain can occur with long-term use.
› Tricyclic antidepressants » Amitriptyline	› Change positions slowly to minimize dizziness from orthostatic hypotension. › To minimize anticholinergic effects, chew sugarless gum, eat foods high in fiber, and increase fluid intake to 2 to 3 L/day from food and beverage sources.
› Monoamine oxidase inhibitors (MAOIs) » Phenelzine (Nardil)	› Due to the risk for hypertensive crisis, avoid foods with tyramine (ripe avocados or figs, fermented or smoked meats, liver, dried or cured fish, most cheeses, some beer and wine, and protein dietary supplements). › Due to the risk of medication interactions, avoid all medications, including over-the-counter, without first discussing them with the provider.
› Atypical antidepressants » Bupropion (Wellbutrin)	› Observe for headache, dry mouth, GI distress, constipation, increased heart rate, nausea, restlessness, or insomnia. Notify the provider if they become intolerable. › Monitor food intake and weight due to appetite suppression. › Avoid administering to clients at risk for seizures.
› Serotonin norepinephrine reuptake inhibitors (SNRIs) » Venlafaxine » Duloxetine (Cymbalta)	› Adverse effects include nausea, weight gain, and sexual dysfunction.

- Teamwork and Collaboration
  - Psychotherapy by a trained therapist can include individual cognitive behavioral therapy (CBT), interpersonal therapy (IPT), group therapy, and family therapy.
    - CBT assists the client to identify and change negative behavior and thought patterns.
    - IPT encourages the client to focus on personal relationships that contribute to the depressive disorder.
- Alternative or Complementary Therapies
  - St. John's wort – A plant product (*Hypericum perforatum*), not regulated by the U.S. Food and Drug Administration, is taken by some individuals to relieve manifestations of mild depression.
    - Nursing Considerations
      - Adverse effects include photosensitivity, skin rash, rapid heart rate, gastrointestinal distress, and abdominal pain.
      - Can increase or reduce levels of some medications if taken concurrently. The client should inform the provider if taking St. John's wort.
      - Medication interactions – Potentially fatal serotonin syndrome can result if taken with SSRIs or other types of antidepressants. Foods containing tyramine should be avoided.
  - Light therapy – First-line treatment for seasonal affective disorder (SAD); inhibits nocturnal secretion of melatonin.
    - Exposure of the face to 10,000-lux light box 30 min a day, once or in two divided doses
- Therapeutic Procedures
  - Electroconvulsive therapy (ECT) can be useful for some clients who have a depressive disorder.
    - Nursing Actions – A specially trained nurse is responsible for monitoring the client before and after this therapy.
  - Transcranial magnetic stimulation (TMS) uses electromagnetic stimulation of the brain. It is indicated for depressive disorders that are resistant to other forms of treatment.
  - Vagus nerve stimulation (VNS) uses an implanted device that stimulates the vagus nerve. It can be used for clients who have depression that is resistant to at least four antidepressant medications.
- Care After Discharge
  - Continuation phase followed by maintenance phase
    - Client Education
      - Review manifestations of depression with the client and family members in order to identify relapse.
      - Reinforce intended effects and potential adverse effects of medication.
      - Explain the benefits of the client's adherence to therapy.

      - Exercise – Thirty minutes of exercise daily for 3 to 5 days each week improves clinical findings of depression and can help to prevent relapse. Even shorter intervals of exercise are helpful. Exercise should be regarded as an adjunct to other therapies for the client who has major depressive disorder.

APPLICATION EXERCISES

1. A nurse working in an acute mental health facility is caring for a 35-year-old female client who has clinical findings of depression. The client lives at home with her husband and two young children. She currently smokes and has a history of chronic asthma. The nurse should identify which of the following as risk factors for depression for this client? (Select all that apply.)

_____ A. Age of 35 years old

_____ B. Female gender

_____ C. History of chronic asthma

_____ D. Currently smokes

_____ E. Being married

2. A nurse working in an outpatient clinic is reinforcing teaching to a client who has a new diagnosis of premenstrual dysphoric disorder (PMDD). Which of the following statements by the client indicates understanding of the teaching?

A. "I can expect my problems with PMDD to be worst when I'm menstruating."

B. "I will use light therapy 30 min a day to prevent further recurrences of PMDD."

C. "I am aware that my PMDD causes me to have rapid mood swings."

D. "I should increase my caloric intake with a nutritional supplement when my PMDD is active."

3. A nurse is discussing the care of a client who has major depressive disorder (MDD) with a newly licensed nurse. Which of the following statements by the newly licensed nurse indicates a need for further reinforcement of teaching?

A. "Care during the continuation phase focuses on treating continued manifestations of MDD."

B. "The goal of treatment during the maintenance phase is prevention of future episodes of MDD."

C. "The client is at greatest risk for suicide during the first weeks of an MDD episode."

D. "Medication and psychotherapy are used to prevent a relapse of MDD."

4. A nurse working on an acute mental health unit is caring for a client who has major depressive disorder and comorbid anxiety disorder. Which of the following is the highest priority action by the nurse?

A. Placing the client on one-to-one observation

B. Assisting the client to perform ADLs

C. Encouraging the client to participate in counseling

D. Telling the client about medication adverse effects

5. A nurse is interviewing a 25-year-old client who has a new diagnosis of dysthymia. Which of the following findings should the nurse expect?

   A. Wide fluctuations in mood

   B. Report of five or more clinical findings of depression

   C. Presence of manifestations for at least 2 years

   D. Inflated sense of self-esteem

6. A nurse working in an acute mental health facility is collecting admission data for a client who has major depressive disorder (MDD). Use the ATI Active Learning Template: Systems Disorder to complete this item to include the following:

   A. Description of Disorder/Disease Process

   B. Data Collection: Objective and Subjective – Identify at least four expected findings.

   C. Patient-Centered Care: Nursing Care – Describe an appropriate communication technique to relate therapeutically with this client.

APPLICATION EXERCISES KEY

1. A. **CORRECT:** Depressive disorders are more prevalent in adults between the ages of 15 and 40.

    B. **CORRECT:** Depressive disorders are twice as common in females than in males.

    C. **CORRECT:** Depressive disorders are more common in clients who have a chronic medical illness.

    D. **CORRECT:** Depressive disorders are more common in clients who have a substance use disorder, such as nicotine use disorder.

    E. INCORRECT: Depressive disorders are more common in unmarried, rather than married, clients.

    Ⓝ NCLEX® Connection: Health Promotion and Maintenance, Health Promotion/Disease Prevention

2. A. INCORRECT: Clinical findings of PMDD are present during the luteal phase of the menstrual cycle, just prior to menses.

    B. INCORRECT: Light therapy is a first-line treatment for seasonal affective disorder, rather than PMDD.

    C. **CORRECT:** A clinical finding of PMDD is emotional lability. The client can experience rapid changes in mood.

    D. INCORRECT: PMDD increases the client's risk for weight gain due to overeating. It is not appropriate to increase caloric intake.

    Ⓝ NCLEX® Connection: Psychosocial Integrity, Therapeutic Communication

3. A. **CORRECT:** The focus of the continuation phase is relapse prevention. Treatment of manifestations occurs during the acute phase of MDD.

    B. INCORRECT: This statement does not indicate a need for further teaching. Prevention of future depressive episodes is the goal of the maintenance phase of treatment.

    C. INCORRECT: This statement does not indicate a need for further teaching. The client is at greatest risk for suicide during the acute phase of MDD.

    D. INCORRECT: This statement does not indicate a need for further teaching. Medication therapy and psychotherapy are used during the continuation phase to prevent relapse of MDD.

    Ⓝ NCLEX® Connection: Psychosocial Integrity, Mental Health Concepts

4.   A. **CORRECT:** The greatest risk for a client who has MDD and comorbid anxiety is injury due to self-harm. The highest priority intervention is placing the client on one-to-one observation.

   B. INCORRECT: The client who has MDD can require assistance with ADLs. However, this does not address the greatest risk to the client and is therefore not the priority intervention.

   C. INCORRECT: The nurse should encourage the client who has MDD to participate in counseling. However, this does not address the greatest risk to the client and is therefore not the priority intervention.

   D. INCORRECT: The nurse should tell the client who has MDD about medication adverse effects. However, this does not address the greatest risk to the client and is therefore not the priority intervention.

   Ⓝ NCLEX® Connection: Psychosocial Integrity, Behavioral Management

5.   A. INCORRECT: Wide fluctuations in mood are associated with bipolar disorder rather than dysthymia.

   B. INCORRECT: MDD, rather than dysthymic disorder, contains a minimum of five clinical findings of depression.

   C. **CORRECT:** The manifestations of dysthymic disorder last for at least 2 years in adults.

   D. INCORRECT: A decreased, rather than inflated, sense of self-esteem is associated with dysthymia.

   Ⓝ NCLEX® Connection: Psychosocial Integrity, Mental Health Concepts

6.   *Using the ATI Active Learning Template: Systems Disorder*

   A. Description of Disorder/Disease Process
   • MDD is a single episode or recurrent episodes of unipolar depression resulting in a significant change in a client's normal functioning (social, occupational, self-care) accompanied by at least five clinical findings of MDD, which must occur almost every day for a minimum of 2 weeks and last most of the day.

   B. Data Collection: Objective and Subjective
   • Depressed mood
   • Difficulty sleeping or excessive sleeping
   • Indecisiveness
   • Decreased ability to concentrate

   • Suicidal ideation
   • Increase or decrease in motor activity
   • Inability to feel pleasure (anhedonia)
   • Increase or decrease in weight of more than 5% of total body weight over 1 month

   C. Patient-Centered Care: Nursing Care
   • Make time to be with the client even if he doesn't speak.
   • Communicate with observations rather than asking direct questions.

   • Give directions in simple, concrete sentences.
   • Allow the client sufficient time to verbally respond.

   Ⓝ NCLEX® Connection: Psychosocial Integrity, Mental Health Concepts

UNIT 3   PSYCHOBIOLOGIC DISORDERS

CHAPTER 13   Bipolar Disorders

Overview

- Bipolar disorders are mood disorders with recurrent episodes of depression and mania.

- Bipolar disorders usually emerge in late adolescence or early adulthood but can be diagnosed in the school-age child. Because the clinical manifestations of bipolar disorder can mimic the expected findings of attention deficit hyperactivity disorder (ADHD), children are more difficult to diagnose than other client age groups.

- Periods of normal functioning alternate with periods of illness, though some clients are not able to maintain full occupational and social functioning.

- Psychotic, paranoid, and/or bizarre behavior can be seen during periods of mania.

- Care of a client who has bipolar disorder mirrors the phase of the disorder the client is experiencing.

PHASE	CHARACTERISTICS	TREATMENT
Acute	› Acute mania	› Hospitalization can be required. › Reduction of mania and client safety are the goals of treatment. › Risk of harm to self or others is determined. › One-to-one supervision can be indicated.
Continuation	› Remission of clinical manifestations	› Treatment is generally 4 to 9 months in duration. › Relapse prevention through education, medication adherence, and psychotherapy is the goal of treatment.
Maintenance	› Increased ability to function	› Treatment generally continues throughout the client's lifetime. › Prevention of future manic episodes is the goal of treatment.

- Behaviors shown with bipolar disorders

  ○ Mania – An abnormally elevated mood, which can be described as expansive or irritable, that usually requires hospitalization. (See the data collection section in this chapter for specific findings.)

  ○ Hypomania – A less severe episode of mania that lasts at least 4 days accompanied by three to four findings of mania. Hospitalization is not required, and the client is less impaired.

  ○ Mixed episode – A manic episode and an episode of major depression experienced simultaneously. The client has marked impairment in functioning and can require admission to an acute care mental health facility to prevent self-harm or other-directed violence.

  ○ Rapid cycling – Four or more episodes of acute mania within 1 year.

- Bipolar disorders recognized and defined by the DSM-5
  - Bipolar I disorder – The client has at least one episode of mania alternating with major depression.
  - Bipolar II disorder – The client has one or more hypomanic episodes alternating with major depressive episodes.
  - Cyclothymia – The client has at least 2 years of repeated hypomanic manifestations that do not meet the criteria for hypomanic episodes alternating with minor depressive episodes.
- Comorbidities associated with bipolar disorder
  - Substance use disorder
    - The client who has a substance use disorder tends to experience more rapid cycling of mania than clients who do not.
    - Substance use is often a means of self-medication. It can have a direct impact on the onset of a mental health disorder, especially if a client is predisposed.
  - Anxiety disorders
  - Eating disorders
  - Attention deficit hyperactivity disorder (ADHD)

 View Video: Understanding Bipolar Disorder

Data Collection

- Risk Factors
  - Genetics, such as having an immediate family member who has a bipolar disorder
  - Psychological, such as stressful events or major life changes
  - Physiological, such as neurobiological and neuroendocrine disorders
  - Substance use disorder, such as alcohol or cocaine use disorder
- Relapse
  - Use of substances (alcohol, cocaine, caffeine) can lead to an episode of mania.
  - Sleep disturbances can come before, be associated with, or be brought on by an episode of mania.
  - Psychological stressors can trigger an episode of mania.

- Subjective and Objective Data

BIPOLAR DISORDER CLINICAL MANIFESTATIONS	
Manic characteristics	
› Labile mood with euphoria	› Demanding and manipulative behavior
› Agitation and irritability	› Distractibility and decreased attention span
› Restlessness	› Poor judgment
› Dislike of interference and intolerance of criticism	› Attention-seeking behavior – flashy dress and makeup, inappropriate behavior
› Increase in talking and activity	› Impairment in social and occupational functioning
› Flight of ideas – rapid, continuous speech with sudden and frequent topic change	› Decreased sleep
› Grandiose view of self and abilities (grandiosity)	› Neglect of ADLs, including nutrition and hydration
› Impulsivity – spending money, giving away money or possessions	› Possible presence of delusions and hallucinations
	› Denial of illness
Depressive characteristics	
› Flat, blunted, labile affect	› Difficulty concentrating, focusing, problem-solving
› Tearfulness, crying	› Self-destructive behavior, including suicidal ideation
› Lack of energy	› Decrease in personal hygiene
› Anhedonia – loss of pleasure and lack of interest in activities, hobbies, sexual activity	› Loss or increase in appetite and/or sleep, disturbed sleep
› Physical reports of discomfort/pain	› Psychomotor retardation or agitation

- Standardized Screening Tool
  - Mood Disorders Questionnaire
    - The Mood Disorders Questionnaire is a standardized tool that places mood progression on a continuum for hypomania (euphoria) to acute mania (extreme irritability and hyperactivity) to delirium (completely out of touch with reality).

Patient-Centered Care

- Nursing Care

  - The care of the client is based on the phase of bipolar disorder that the client is experiencing. Nursing care is provided throughout this process.

  - Acute Manic Episode

    - Focus is on safety and maintaining physical health.

    - Therapeutic milieu (within acute care mental health facility)

      □ Provide a safe environment during the acute phase.

      □ Monitor the client regularly for suicidal thoughts, intentions, and escalating behavior.

      □ Decrease stimulation without isolating the client if possible. Be aware of noise, music, television, and other clients, all of which can lead to an escalation of the client's behavior. In certain cases, seclusion can be the only way to safely decrease stimulation for the client.

      □ Follow agency protocols for providing client protection (restraints, seclusion, one-to-one observation) if a threat of self-injury or injury to others exists.

      □ Implement frequent rest periods.

      □ Provide outlets for physical activity. Do not involve the client in activities that last a long time or that require a high level of concentration and/or detailed instructions.

      □ Protect client from poor judgment and impulsive behavior, such as giving money away and sexual indiscretions.

      □ Maintenance of self-care needs

        ‣ Monitor sleep, fluid intake, and nutrition.

        ‣ Provide portable, nutritious food because the client might not be able to sit down to eat.

        ‣ Supervise choice of clothes.

        ‣ Give step-by-step reminders for hygiene and dress.

      □ Communication

        ‣ Use a calm, matter-of-fact, specific approach.

        ‣ Give concise explanations.

        ‣ Provide for consistency with expectations and limit-setting.

        ‣ Avoid power struggles, and do not react personally to the client's comments.

        ‣ Listen to and act on legitimate client grievances.

        ‣ Reinforce nonmanipulative behaviors.

- Medications
  - Mood stabilizers
    - Lithium carbonate (Lithobid)
    - Anticonvulsants that act as mood stabilizers, including valproic acid (Depakote), clonazepam (Klonopin), lamotrigine (Lamictal), gabapentin (Neurontin), and topiramate (Topamax)
  - Benzodiazepines, such as lorazepam (Ativan), used on a short-term basis for a client experiencing sleep impairment related to mania
  - Antidepressants, such as the SSRI fluoxetine (Prozac), used to manage a major depressive episode
- Therapeutic Procedures
  - Electroconvulsive therapy (ECT)
    - Electroconvulsive therapy (ECT) can be used to subdue extreme manic behavior, especially when pharmacologic therapy, such as lithium, has not worked. ECT also can be used for clients who are suicidal or who have rapid cycling.

- Client Education
  - Case management to provide follow-up for the client the family
  - Group, family, and individual psychotherapy to improve problem-solving and interpersonal skills
  - Health teaching to reinforce
    - The chronicity of the disorder requiring long-term pharmacological and psychological support
    - The benefits of psychotherapy and support groups to prevent relapse
    - Indications of impending relapse and ways to manage the crisis
    - Precipitating factors of relapse (e.g., sleep disturbance; use of alcohol, caffeine, or drugs of abuse)
    - The importance of maintaining a regular sleep, meal, and activity pattern
    - Medication administration and adherence

Complications

- Physical exhaustion and possible death
  - A client in a true manic state usually will not stop moving, and does not eat, drink, or sleep. This can become a medical emergency.
  - Nursing Actions
    - Prevent client self-harm.
    - Decrease the client's physical activity.
    - Ensure adequate fluid and food intake.
    - Promote an adequate amount of sleep each night.
    - Assist the client with self-care needs.
    - Manage medication appropriately.

APPLICATION EXERCISES

1. A nurse is assisting with planning care for a client who has bipolar disorder and is experiencing a manic episode. Which of the following are appropriate nursing interventions? (Select all that apply.)

_____ A. Provide flexible client behavior expectations

_____ B. Offer concise explanations

_____ C. Establish consistent limits

_____ D. Disregard client complaints

_____ E. Use a firm approach with communication

2. A nurse is assisting with conducting an in-service about the use of electroconvulsive therapy (ECT) for the treatment of bipolar disorder. Which of the following statements by a newly licensed nurse indicates understanding?

A. "ECT is the recommended initial treatment for bipolar disorder."

B. "ECT is contraindicated for clients who have suicidal ideation."

C. "ECT is effective for clients who are experiencing severe mania."

D. "ECT is prescribed to prevent relapse of bipolar disorder."

3. A nurse in an acute mental health facility is caring for a client who is experiencing a mixed episode of bipolar disorder. Which of the following is the priority nursing action?

A. Set consistent limits for expected client behavior.

B. Administer prescribed medications as scheduled.

C. Provide the client with step-by-step instructions during hygiene activities.

D. Monitor the client for escalating behavior.

4. A nurse is caring for a client who has bipolar disorder. The client states, "I am very rich, and I feel I must give my money to you." Which of the following is an appropriate response by the nurse?

A. "Why do you think you feel the need to give money away?"

B. "I am here to provide care and cannot accept this from you."

C. "I can request that your case manager discuss appropriate charity options with you."

D. "You should know that giving away your money is inappropriate."

5. A nurse is reinforcing teaching regarding relapse prevention with a client who has bipolar disorder. Which of the following should the nurse include in the discussion? (Select all that apply.)

_____ A. Use caffeine in moderation to prevent relapse.

_____ B. Difficulty sleeping can indicate a relapse.

_____ C. Begin taking your medications as soon as a relapse begins.

_____ D. Participating in psychotherapy can help prevent a relapse.

_____ E. Anhedonia is a clinical manifestation of a depressive relapse.

6. A nurse in an acute mental health facility is caring for a client who is experiencing acute mania. Use the ATI Active Learning Template: Systems Disorder to complete this item to include the following:

A. Description of Disorder/Disease Process

B. Data Collection: Objective and Subjective – Identify two expected findings.

C. Collaborative Care: Nursing Care – Identify two nursing actions.

APPLICATION EXERCISES KEY

1. A. INCORRECT: The nurse should establish consistent client behavior expectations to decrease the risk for client manipulation.

   B. **CORRECT:** Offering concise explanations improves the client's ability to focus and comprehend the information.

   C. **CORRECT:** Establishing consistent limits decreases the risk for client manipulation.

   D. INCORRECT: The nurse should respond to valid client complaints to foster a trusting nurse-client relationship.

   E. **CORRECT:** Using a firm approach with client communication promotes structure and minimizes inappropriate client behaviors.

   Ⓝ NCLEX® Connection: Psychosocial Integrity, Behavioral Management

2. A. INCORRECT: Pharmacological intervention is the recommended initial treatment for bipolar disorder.

   B. INCORRECT: ECT is effective for clients who have bipolar disorder and suicidal ideation.

   C. **CORRECT:** ECT is appropriate for the treatment of severe mania associated with bipolar disorder.

   D. INCORRECT: ECT is prescribed for clients experiencing an acute episode of bipolar disorder rather than for the prevention of relapse.

   Ⓝ NCLEX® Connection: Reduction of Risk Potential, Potential for Complications of Diagnostic Tests/Treatments/Procedures

3. A. INCORRECT: Setting consistent limits for expected client behavior is appropriate. However, this does not address the client's priority need for safety and is therefore not the priority action.

   B. INCORRECT: Administering prescribed medications as scheduled is appropriate. However, this does not address the client's priority need for safety and is therefore not the priority action.

   C. INCORRECT: Providing the client with step-by-step instructions during hygiene activities is appropriate. However, this does not address the client's priority need for safety and is therefore not the priority action.

   D. **CORRECT:** Monitoring the client for escalating behavior addresses the client's priority need for safety and is therefore the priority nursing action.

   Ⓝ NCLEX® Connection: Psychosocial Integrity, Mental Health Concepts

4. A. INCORRECT: Asking a "why" question is a nontherapeutic form of communication and can promote a defensive client response.

   B. **CORRECT:** This statement is matter-of-fact and concise and is an appropriate response to a client who has bipolar disorder.

   C. INCORRECT: This statement does not recognize the possibility of poor judgment, which is associated with bipolar disorder.

   D. INCORRECT: This statement offers disapproval and can be interpreted by the client as aggressive, which can promote a defensive client response.

   Ⓝ NCLEX® Connection: Psychosocial Integrity, Therapeutic Communication

5. A. INCORRECT: The client who has bipolar disorder should avoid the use of caffeine because it can precipitate a relapse.

    B. **CORRECT:** The client should be alert for sleep disturbances, which can indicate a relapse.

    C. INCORRECT: The client who has bipolar disorder should take prescribed medications to prevent and minimize a relapse.

    D. **CORRECT:** The client who has bipolar disorder can participate in psychotherapy to help prevent a relapse.

    E. **CORRECT:** The client who has bipolar disorder should be aware of clinical manifestations, including anhedonia, which is a depressive characteristic that can indicate a relapse.

    Ⓝ NCLEX® Connection: Psychosocial Integrity, Mental Health Concepts

6. *Using the ATI Active Learning Template: Systems Disorder*

    A. Description of Disorder/Disease Process
       • An abnormally elevated mood, which can be described as expansive or irritable, that usually requires hospitalization

    B. Data Collection: Objective and Subjective
       • Agitation and irritability
       • Intolerance of interference or criticism
       • Increase in talking and activity
       • Flight of ideas
       • Grandiosity
       • Impulsivity
       • Demanding and manipulative behavior
       • Distractibility
       • Poor judgment
       • Attention-seeking behavior
       • Impairment in social and occupational functioning
       • Decreased sleep
       • Neglect of ADLs
       • Possible delusions and hallucinations
       • Denial of illness

    C. Collaborative Care: Nursing Care
       • Focus on safety as the priority of care.
       • Maintain the client's physical health and self-care needs.
       • Provide a safe environment.
       • Check for suicidal thoughts, intentions, and escalating behavior.
       • Decrease stimulation.
       • Provide client protection with restraints, seclusion, or one-to-one observation if necessary.
       • Implement frequent rest periods.
       • Provide appropriate outlets for physical activity.
       • Use calm and concise communication.

    Ⓝ NCLEX® Connection: Psychosocial Integrity, Mental Health Concepts

chapter **14**

Overview

- Schizophrenia spectrum and other psychotic disorders affect thinking, behavior, emotions, and the ability to perceive reality.

- Schizophrenia probably results from a combination of genetic, neurobiological, and nongenetic (injury at birth, viral infection, and nutritional) factors.

- The typical age at onset is late teens and early 20s, but schizophrenia has occurred in young children and may begin in later adulthood.

- A diagnosis of schizophrenia should not be made for children until after age 7 to rule out attention deficit hyperactivity disorder (ADHD) with violent tendencies.

- Psychotic disorders become problematic when manifestations interfere with interpersonal relationships, self-care, and ability to work.

- The various types of psychotic disorders recognized and defined by the DSM-5 include the following.

  - Schizophrenia – The client has psychotic thinking or behavior present for at least 6 months. Areas of functioning, including school or work, self-care, and interpersonal relationships, are significantly impaired.

  - Schizotypal personality disorder – The client has impairments of personality (self and interpersonal) functioning. However, impairment is not as severe as with schizophrenia.

  - Delusional disorder – The client experiences delusional thinking for at least 1 month. Self or interpersonal functioning is not markedly impaired.

  - Brief psychotic disorder – The client has psychotic manifestations that last between 1 day to 1 month in duration.

  - Schizophreniform disorder – The client has manifestations similar to those of schizophrenia, but the duration is from 1 to 6 months, and social/occupational dysfunction may or may not be present.

  - Schizoaffective disorder – The client's disorder meets both the criteria for schizophrenia and depressive or bipolar disorder.

  - Substance-induced psychotic disorder – The client experiences psychosis within 1 month of substance intoxication or withdrawal. Can be caused by medications intended for therapeutic use.

Data Collection

- Subjective and Objective Data

CHARACTERISTIC DIMENSIONS OF PSYCHOTIC DISORDERS	
Positive symptoms – The manifestation of things that are not normally present. These are the most easily identified symptoms.	
› Hallucinations	› Alterations in speech
› Delusions	› Bizarre behavior, such as walking backward constantly
Negative symptoms – The absence of things that are normally present. These symptoms are more difficult to treat successfully than positive symptoms.	
› Affect – usually blunted (narrow range of normal expression) or flat (facial expression never changes) › Alogia – poverty of thought or speech; the client might sit with a visitor but only mumble or respond vaguely to questions. › Anergia – lack of energy	› Anhedonia – lack of pleasure or joy; the client is indifferent to things that often make others happy, such as looking at beautiful scenery. › Avolition – lack of motivation in activities and hygiene; for example, the client completes an assigned task, such as making his bed, but is unable to start the next common chore without prompting.
Cognitive manifestations – Problems with thinking make it very difficult for the client to live independently.	
› Disordered thinking › Inability to make decisions › Poor problem-solving ability › Difficulty concentrating to perform tasks	› Memory deficits » Long-term memory » Working memory, such as inability to follow directions to find an address
Affective manifestations – Manifestations involving emotions.	
› Hopelessness	› Suicidal ideation

- Alterations in thought (delusions) are false fixed beliefs that cannot be corrected by reasoning and are usually bizarre. These include the following.

DELUSIONS	EXAMPLES
Ideas of reference	› Misconstrues trivial events and attaches personal significance to them, such as believing that others, who are discussing the next meal, are talking about him.
Persecution	› Feels singled out for harm by others (e.g., being hunted down by the FBI).
Grandeur	› Believes that she is all powerful and important, like a god.
Somatic delusions	› Believes that his body is changing in an unusual way, such as growing a third arm.
Jealousy	› May feel that her spouse is sexually involved with another individual.
Being controlled	› Believes that a force outside his body is controlling him.
Thought broadcasting	› Believes that her thoughts are heard by others.
Thought insertion	› Believes that others' thoughts are being inserted into his mind.
Thought withdrawal	› Believes that her thoughts have been removed from her mind by an outside agency.
Religiosity	› Is obsessed with religious beliefs.

○ Following are examples of alterations in speech that can occur.

ALTERATIONS IN SPEECH	
Flight of ideas	› Associative looseness
	› The client might say sentence after sentence, but each sentence relates to another topic, and the listener is unable to follow the client's thoughts.
Neologisms	› Made-up words that have meaning only to the client, such as, "I tranged and flittled."
Echolalia	› The client repeats the words spoken to him.
Clang association	› Meaningless rhyming of words, often forceful, such as, "Oh fox, box, and lox."
Word salad	› Words jumbled together with little meaning or significance to the listener, such as, "Hip hooray, the flip is cast and wide-sprinting in the forest."

○ Alterations in perception

■ Hallucinations are sensory perceptions that do not have any apparent external stimulus. Examples include the following.

□ Auditory – hearing voices or sounds

▶ Command – The voice instructs the client to perform an action, such as to hurt self or others.

□ Visual – seeing persons or things

□ Olfactory – smelling odors

□ Gustatory – experiencing tastes

□ Tactile – feeling bodily sensations

■ Personal boundary difficulties – disenfranchisement with one's own body, identity, and perceptions. This includes the following.

□ Depersonalization – nonspecific feeling that a person has lost her identity; self is different or unreal

□ Derealization – perception that environment has changed

■ Alterations in behavior

□ Extreme agitation, including pacing and rocking

□ Stereotyped behaviors – motor patterns that had meaning to client (sweeping the floor) but now are mechanical and lack purpose

□ Automatic obedience – responding in a robotlike manner

□ Wavy flexibility – excessive maintenance of position

□ Stupor – motionless for long periods of time, comalike

□ Negativism – doing the opposite of what is requested

□ Echopraxia – purposeful imitation of movements made by others

• Standardized Screening Tools

○ The Global Assessment of Functioning (GAF) scale – This scale helps to determine a client's ability to perform activities of daily living and to function independently. The GAF is appropriate for use with all clients who have a mental health disorder.

○ Scale for Assessment of Negative Symptoms

○ Brief Psychiatric Rating Scale (BPRS)

○ Abnormal Involuntary Movement Scale (AIMS)

Patient-Centered Care

- Nursing Care

    - Milieu therapy is used for clients who have a psychotic disorder both in acute mental health facilities and in community facilities, such as residential crisis centers, halfway houses, and day treatment programs.

        - Provide a structured, safe environment (milieu) for the client in order to decrease anxiety and to distract the client from constant thinking about hallucinations.

        - Assertive community treatment (ACT) – intensive case management and interprofessional team approach to assist clients with community-living needs.

    - Promote therapeutic communication to lower anxiety, decrease defensive patterns, and encourage participation in the milieu.

    - Establish a trusting relationship with the client.

    - Encourage the development of social skills and friendships.

    - Encourage participation in group work and psychoeducation.

    - Use appropriate communication to address hallucinations and delusions.

        - Ask the client directly about hallucinations. The nurse should not argue or agree with the client's view of the situation, but may offer a comment, such as, "I don't hear anything, but you seem to be feeling frightened."

        - Do not argue with a client's delusions, but focus on the client's feelings and possibly offer reasonable explanations, such as, "I can't imagine that the president of the United States would have a reason to kill a citizen, but it must be frightening for you to believe that."

        - Monitor the client for paranoid delusions, which can increase the risk for violence against others.

        - Provide for safety if the client is experiencing command hallucinations due to the increased risk for harm to self or others.

        - Attempt to focus conversations on reality-based subjects.

        - Identify symptom triggers, such as loud noises (can trigger auditory hallucinations in some clients) and situations that seem to trigger conversations about the client's delusions.

        - Be genuine and empathetic in all dealings with the client.

    - Collect data about the client's discharge needs, such as ability to perform activities of daily living.

    - Promote self-care by modeling and reinforcing self-care activities within the mental health facility.

    - Relate wellness to the elements of symptom management.

    - Collaborate with the client to use symptom management techniques to cope with depressive manifestations and anxiety. Symptom management techniques include strategies such as using music to distract from "voices," attending activities, walking, talking to a trusted person when hallucinations are most bothersome, and interacting with an auditory or visual hallucination by telling it to stop or go away.

    - Encourage medication compliance.

    - Reinforce teaching regarding medications.

    - Whenever possible, incorporate family in all aspects of care.

MEDICATIONS FOR PSYCHOTIC DISORDERS	EXAMPLES OF MEDICATION	NURSING INTERVENTIONS/CLIENT EDUCATION
› Atypical antipsychotics are current medications of choice for psychotic disorders, and they generally treat both positive and negative symptoms.	› Risperidone (Risperdal) › Olanzapine (Zyprexa) › Quetiapine (Seroquel) › Ziprasidone (Geodon) › Aripiprazole (Abilify) › Clozapine (Clozaril)	› To minimize weight gain, advise the client to follow a healthy, low-calorie diet, engage in regular exercise, and monitor weight. › Manifestations of agitation, dizziness, sedation, and sleep disruption can occur. Instruct the client to report these adverse effects because the provider may need to change the medication.
› Conventional antipsychotics are used to treat mainly positive psychotic symptoms.	› Haloperidol (Haldol) › Loxapine › Chlorpromazine › Fluphenazine	› To minimize anticholinergic effects, advise the client to chew gum, eat foods high in fiber, and eat and drink 2 to 3 L of fluid a day from food and beverage sources. › Instruct the client about indications of postural hypotension (e.g., lightheadedness, dizziness). If these occur, advise the client to sit or lie down. Minimize orthostatic hypotension by getting up slowly from a lying or sitting position.
› Antidepressants are used to treat the depression seen in many clients who have a psychotic disorder.	› Paroxetine (Paxil)	› Used temporarily to treat depression associated with psychotic disorders. › Monitor for suicidal ideation because this medication can increase thoughts of self-harm, especially when first taking it. › Notify the provider of any adverse effects, such as deepened depression. › Advise the client to avoid abrupt cessation of this medication to avoid a withdrawal effect.
› Anxiolytics/benzodiazepines are used to treat the anxiety often found in clients who have psychotic disorders, as well as some of the positive and negative symptoms.	› Lorazepam (Ativan) › Clonazepam (Klonopin)	› Inform the client of this medication's sedative effects. › Inform the client of the need for blood tests to monitor for agranulocytosis. › These medications are used with caution in older adult clients.

- Care After Discharge
  - Client Education

    - Case management to provide follow up for the client and family.
    - Group, family, and individual psychoeducation to improve problem-solving and interpersonal skills.
    - Social skills training focuses on reinforcing social and ADL skills.
    - Reinforce health teaching regarding the following.
      - Understanding of the disorder
      - Need for self-care to prevent relapse
      - Medication effects, adverse effects, and importance of compliance
      - Importance of attending support groups
      - Abstinence from the use of alcohol and drugs
      - Keeping a log or journal of feelings and changes in behavior to help monitor medication effectiveness

APPLICATION EXERCISES

1. A nurse is caring for a client who has substance-induced psychotic disorder and is experiencing auditory hallucinations. The client states, "The voices won't leave me alone!" Which of the following statements by the nurse are appropriate? (Select all that apply.)

_____ A. "When did you start hearing the voices?"

_____ B. "The voices are not real, or else we would both hear them."

_____ C. "It must be scary to hear voices."

_____ D. "Are the voices telling you to hurt yourself?"

_____ E. "Why are the voices talking to only you?"

2. A nurse is collecting data on a client who has schizophrenia. Which of the following findings should the nurse document as positive symptoms? (Select all that apply.)

_____ A. Auditory hallucination

_____ B. Lack of motivation

_____ C. Use of clang associations

_____ D. Delusion of persecution

_____ E. Constantly waving arms

_____ F. Flat affect

3. A nurse is caring for a client who has schizoaffective disorder. Which of the following statements indicates the client is experiencing depersonalization?

A. "I am a superhero and am immortal."

B. "I am no one, and everyone is me."

C. "I feel monsters pinching me all over."

D. "I know that you are stealing my thoughts."

4. A nurse is speaking with a client who has schizophrenia when he suddenly seems to stop focusing on the nurse's questions and begins looking at the ceiling and talking to himself. Which of the following actions should the nurse take?

  A. Stop the interview at this point, and resume later when the client is better able to concentrate.

  B. Ask the client, "Are you seeing something on the ceiling?"

  C. Tell the client, "You seem to be looking at something on the ceiling. I see something there, too."

  D. Continue the interview without comment on the client's behavior.

5. A nurse is caring for a client on an acute mental health unit. The client reports hearing voices that are telling her to "kill your doctor." Which of the following is the priority action for the nurse to take?

  A. Use therapeutic communication to discuss the hallucination with the client.

  B. Initiate one-to-one observation of the client.

  C. Focus the client on reality.

  D. Notify the provider of the client's statement.

6. A nurse is caring for a client who has schizophrenia and is reinforcing discharge instructions that include a new prescription for risperidone (Risperdal). Use the ATI Active Learning Template: Medication and the ATI Pharmacology Review Module to complete the following:

  A. Therapeutic Use

  B. Nursing Interventions/Client Education: Describe at least three.

APPLICATION EXERCISES KEY

1. A. **CORRECT:** The nurse should ask the client directly about the hallucination.

    B. INCORRECT: The nurse should not argue with the client's view of the situation.

    C. **CORRECT:** The nurse should focus on the client's feelings rather than agreeing with the client's hallucination.

    D. **CORRECT:** The nurse should collect data about the presence of command hallucinations and the client's risk for injury to self or others.

    E. INCORRECT: The nurse should avoid asking a "why" question, which is nontherapeutic and can promote a defensive client response.

    Ⓝ NCLEX® Connection: Psychosocial Integrity, Sensory/Perceptual Alterations

2. A. **CORRECT:** Hallucinations are an example of a positive symptom.

    B. INCORRECT: Lack of motivation, or avolition, is an example of a negative symptom.

    C. **CORRECT:** Alterations in speech are an example of a positive symptom.

    D. **CORRECT:** Delusions are an example of a positive symptom.

    E. **CORRECT:** Bizarre motor movements are an example of a positive symptom.

    F. INCORRECT: Flat affect is an example of a negative symptom.

    Ⓝ NCLEX® Connection: Psychosocial Integrity, Mental Health Concepts

3. A. INCORRECT: This comment indicates the client is experiencing delusions of grandeur rather than depersonalization.

    B. **CORRECT:** This comment indicates the client is experiencing a loss of identity or depersonalization.

    C. INCORRECT: This comment indicates the client is experiencing a tactile hallucination rather than depersonalization.

    D. INCORRECT: This comment indicates the client is experiencing thought withdrawal rather than depersonalization.

    Ⓝ NCLEX® Connection: Psychosocial Integrity, Mental Health Concepts

4. A. INCORRECT: The nurse should address the client's current needs related to the possible hallucination rather than stop the interview.

    B. **CORRECT:** The nurse should ask the client directly about the hallucination to identify client needs and check for a potential risk for injury.

    C. INCORRECT: The nurse should avoid agreeing with the client, which can promote psychotic thinking.

    D. INCORRECT: The nurse should address the client's current needs related to the possible hallucination rather than ignoring the change in behavior.

    Ⓝ NCLEX® Connection: Psychosocial Integrity, Sensory/Perceptual Alterations

5. A. INCORRECT: It is appropriate for the nurse to use therapeutic communication to discuss the client's hallucination. However, this does not address the issue of client safety and is therefore not the priority action.

    B. **CORRECT:** A client who is experiencing a command hallucination is at risk for injury to self or others. Therefore, safety is the priority, and initiating one-to-one observation is the priority action.

    C. INCORRECT: It is appropriate for the nurse to attempt to focus the client on reality. However, this does not address the issue of client safety and is therefore not the priority action.

    D. INCORRECT: It is appropriate for the nurse to notify the provider of the client's hallucination. However, this does not address the issue of client safety and is therefore not the priority action.

    Ⓝ NCLEX® Connection: Psychosocial Integrity, Crisis Intervention

6. *Using the ATI Active Learning Template: Medication*

    A. Therapeutic Use
    - Risperidone is an atypical antipsychotic used to treat positive, negative, and affective symptoms of schizophrenia.

    B. Nursing Interventions/Client Education
    - Advise the client to follow a healthy, low-calorie diet.
    - Recommend regular exercise.
    - Instruct the client to monitor weight.
    - Reinforce teaching about adverse effects and instruct the client to notify the provider if these effects are present.
    - Risperidone has a lower risk of extrapyramidal side effects than typical antipsychotics.
    - Risperidone has a lower risk of anticholinergic adverse effects than typical antipsychotics.

    Ⓝ NCLEX® Connection: Pharmacological Therapies, Expected Actions/Outcomes

chapter 15

Overview

- A client who has a personality disorder demonstrates pathological personality characteristics.

- A client who has a personality disorder exhibits impairments in self-identity or self-direction and interpersonal functioning.

- The maladaptive behaviors of a personality disorder are not always perceived by the individual as dysfunctional. Some areas of personal functioning can be adequate.

- Personality disorders often co-occur with other mental health diagnoses, such as depression, anxiety, eating disorders, and substance use disorders.

- Defense mechanisms used by clients who have personality disorders include repression, suppression, regression, undoing, and splitting.

  - Splitting, which is the inability to incorporate positive and negative aspects of oneself or others into a whole image, is frequently seen in the acute mental health setting.

  - Splitting is commonly associated with borderline personality disorder.

  - In splitting, the client tends to characterize people or things as all good or all bad at any particular moment. For example, the client might say, "You are the worst person in the world." Later that day, she might say, "You are the best, but the nurse from the last shift is absolutely terrible."

Data Collection

- Risk Factors

  - Comorbid substance use disorders

  - History of nonviolent and violent crimes, including sex offenses

  - Psychosocial influences, such as childhood abuse or trauma

  - Developmental factors with a direct link to parenting

  - Biological influences, including genetic and biochemical factors

- Subjective and Objective Data

  - Clients who have a personality disorder will exhibit one or more of the following common pathological personality characteristics.

    - Inflexibility/maladaptive responses to stress

    - Compulsiveness and lack of social restraint

    - Inability to emotionally connect in social and professional relationships

    - Tendency to provoke interpersonal conflict

    - Ability to merge personal boundaries with others

THE 10 PERSONALITY DISORDERS	
CLUSTER A (ODD OR ECCENTRIC TRAITS)	
Paranoid	› Characterized by distrust and suspiciousness toward others based on unfounded beliefs that others want to harm, exploit, or deceive the person
Schizoid	› Characterized by emotional detachment, disinterest in close relationships, and indifference to praise or criticism › Often uncooperative
Schizotypal	› Characterized by odd beliefs leading to interpersonal difficulties, an eccentric appearance, and magical thinking or perceptual distortions that are not clear delusions or hallucinations
CLUSTER B (DRAMATIC, EMOTIONAL, OR ERRATIC TRAITS)	
Antisocial	› Characterized by disregard for others with exploitation, repeated unlawful actions, deceit, and failure to accept personal responsibility
Borderline	› Characterized by instability of affect, identity, and relationships, as well as splitting behaviors, manipulation, impulsiveness, and fear of abandonment › Often tries self-injury and can be suicidal
Histrionic	› Characterized by emotional attention-seeking behavior, in which the person needs to be the center of attention › Often seductive and flirtatious
Narcissistic	› Characterized by arrogance, grandiose views of self-importance, the need for consistent admiration, and a lack of empathy for others that strains most relationships › Often sensitive to criticism
CLUSTER C (ANXIOUS OR FEARFUL TRAITS; INSECURITY AND INADEQUACY)	
Avoidant	› Characterized by social inhibition and avoidance of all situations that require interpersonal contact, despite wanting close relationships, due to extreme fear of rejection › Often very anxious in social situations
Dependent	› Characterized by extreme dependency in a close relationship with an urgent search to find a replacement when one relationship ends
Obsessive-compulsive	› Characterized by perfectionism with a focus on orderliness and control to the extent that the individual might not be able to accomplish a given task

Patient-Centered Care

- Nursing Care
  - Self-assessment is vital for nurses caring for clients who have personality disorders and should be performed prior to care.
    - Clients who have personality disorder can evoke intense emotions in the nurse.
    - Awareness of personal reactions to stress promotes effective nursing care.
    - Therapeutic communication and intervention are promoted when client behaviors are anticipated.
    - The nurse should repeat the self-assessment if experiencing a personal stress response to client behavior.

- ○ Milieu management focuses on appropriate social interaction within a group context.
- ○ Safety is always a priority concern because some clients who have a personality disorder are at risk for self-injury or violence.
- ○ Communication strategies
  - Developing a therapeutic relationship is often challenging due to the client's distrust or hostility toward others. Feelings of being threatened or having no control can cause a client to act out toward the nurse.
    - □ A firm, yet supportive approach and consistent care will help build a therapeutic nurse-client relationship.
    - □ Offer the client realistic choices to enhance the client's sense of control.

    - □ Limit-setting and consistency are essential with clients who are manipulative, especially those who have borderline or antisocial personality disorders.
    - □ Clients who have dependent and histrionic personality disorders often benefit from assertiveness training and modeling.
    - □ Clients who have schizoid or schizotypal personality disorders tend to isolate themselves. The nurse should respect this need.
    - □ For clients who have histrionic personality disorder and can be flirtatious, it is important for the nurse to maintain professional boundaries and communication at all times.
    - □ When caring for clients who exhibit dependent behavior, self-assess frequently for countertransference reactions.
- • Medications
  - ○ Medications include the use of psychotropic agents to provide relief from clinical manifestations.
  - ○ Antidepressant, anxiolytic, antipsychotic, or mood stabilizer medications can be prescribed.
- • Teamwork and Collaboration
  - ○ Psychobiological interventions include the following.
    - Psychotherapy, group therapy, and cognitive behavioral therapy are effective treatment modalities for clients who have personality disorders.
    - Dialectical behavior therapy is a cognitive behavioral therapy used for clients who exhibit self-injurious behavior. It focuses on gradual behavior changes and provides acceptance and validation for these clients.
    - Case management is beneficial for clients who have personality disorders and are persistently and severely impaired.
      - □ In acute care facilities, case management focuses on obtaining pertinent history from current or previous providers, supporting reintegration with the family, and ensuring appropriate referrals to outpatient care.
      - □ In long-term outpatient facilities, case management goals include reducing hospitalization by providing resources for crisis services and enhancing the social support system.

APPLICATION EXERCISES

1. A nurse is discussing the care of a client who has a personality disorder with a newly licensed nurse. Which of the following statements by the newly licensed nurse indicates a need for further teaching?

    A. "I can promote my client's sense of control by establishing a schedule."

    B. "Self-assessment will help me cope with emotional reactions to client care."

    C. "I should practice limit-setting to help prevent client manipulation."

    D. "Maintaining professional boundaries is a priority of client care."

2. A nurse is caring for a client who has avoidant personality disorder. Which of the following statements is expected from a client who has this type of personality disorder?

    A. "I'm scared that you're going to leave me."

    B. "I'll go to group therapy if you'll let me smoke."

    C. "I need to feel that everyone admires me."

    D. "I sometimes feel better if I cut myself."

3. A nurse is assisting with the preparation of a staff education session on personality disorders. Which of the following should be included as personality characteristics associated with all personality disorders? (Select all that apply.)

    _____ A. Difficulty in getting along with other members of a group

    _____ B. Belief in the ability to become invisible during times of stress

    _____ C. Display of defense mechanisms when routines are changed

    _____ D. Claiming to be more important than other persons

    _____ E. Difficulty understanding why it is inappropriate to have a personal relationship with staff

4. A nurse is caring for a client who has borderline personality disorder. The client says, "The nurse on the evening shift is always nice! You are the meanest nurse ever!" The nurse should recognize the client's statement as an example of which of the following defense mechanisms?

    A. Regression

    B. Splitting

    C. Undoing

    D. Identification

5. A nurse is assisting with a court-ordered evaluation of a client who has antisocial personality disorder. When collecting data on this client, which of the following are expected findings? (Select all that apply.)

_____ A. Demonstrates extreme anxiety when placed in a social situation

_____ B. Has difficulty making even simple decisions

_____ C. Attempts to convince other clients to give him their belongings

_____ D. Becomes agitated if his personal area is not neat and orderly

_____ E. Blames others for his past and current problems

6. A nurse is discussing self-assessment with a newly licensed nurse. Use the ATI Active Learning Template: Basic Concept to complete this item to include:

A. Related Content: Identify how self-assessment relates to caring for a client who has a personality disorder.

B. Underlying Principles: Identify at least two concepts.

C. Nursing Interventions: Identify who should perform self-assessment and when it is indicated.

APPLICATION EXERCISES KEY

1. A. **CORRECT:** Rather than establishing a schedule, the nurse should ask for the client's input and offer realistic choices to promote the client's sense of control.

    B. INCORRECT: Caring for a client who has a personality disorder can evoke an intense emotional response by the nurse. Self-assessment assists the nurse to cope with these reactions.

    C. INCORRECT: When caring for a client who has a personality disorder, limit-setting is appropriate to help prevent client manipulation.

    D. INCORRECT: When caring for a client who has a personality disorder, the nurse should always maintain professional boundaries.

    Ⓝ NCLEX® Connection: Psychosocial Integrity, Mental Health Concepts

2. A. **CORRECT:** Clients who have avoidant personality disorder often have a fear of abandonment. This type of statement is expected.

    B. INCORRECT: This statement indicates manipulation, which is not expected from a client who has borderline personality disorder.

    C. INCORRECT: This statement indicates a need for admiration, which is expected from a client who has narcissistic personality disorder.

    D. INCORRECT: This statement indicates a risk for self-injury, which is expected from a client who has borderline personality disorder.

    Ⓝ NCLEX® Connection: Psychosocial Integrity, Mental Health Concepts

3. A. **CORRECT:** Difficulty with social and professional relationships is a personality characteristic that can be seen with all personality disorder types.

    B. INCORRECT: Clients who have schizotypal personality disorder can display magical thinking or delusions. However, this is not associated with all personality disorder types.

    C. **CORRECT:** Maladaptive response to stress is a personality characteristic that can be seen with all personality disorder types.

    D. INCORRECT: Clients who have narcissistic personality disorder can display grandiose thinking. However, this is not associated with all personality disorder types.

    E. **CORRECT:** Difficulty understanding personal boundaries is a personality characteristic that can be seen with all personality disorder types.

    Ⓝ NCLEX® Connection: Psychosocial Integrity, Mental Health Concepts

4. A. INCORRECT: Regression refers to resorting to an earlier way of functioning, such as having a temper tantrum.

    B. **CORRECT:** Splitting occurs when a person is unable to see both positive and negative qualities at the same time. The client who has borderline personality disorder tends to see a person as all bad one time and all good another time.

    C. INCORRECT: Undoing is a behavior that is intended to undo or reverse unacceptable thoughts or acts, such as buying a gift for a spouse after having an extramarital affair.

    D. INCORRECT: In identification, the person imitates the behavior of someone admired or feared.

    Ⓝ NCLEX® Connection: Psychosocial Integrity, Mental Health Concepts

5. A. INCORRECT: Anxiety in social situations is an expected finding of clients who have avoidant rather than antisocial personality disorder.

    B. INCORRECT: Indecisiveness, due to a sensitivity to criticism, is an expected finding of clients who have narcissistic rather than antisocial personality disorder.

    C. **CORRECT:** Exploitation and manipulation of others is an expected finding of antisocial personality disorder.

    D. INCORRECT: Perfectionism with a focus on orderliness and control is an expected finding of clients who have obsessive-compulsive rather than antisocial personality disorder.

    E. **CORRECT:** Failure to accept personal responsibility is an expected finding of clients who have antisocial personality disorder.

    Ⓝ NCLEX® Connection: Psychosocial Integrity, Mental Health Concepts

6. *Using the ATI Active Learning Template: Basic Concept*

    A. Related Content
    - Self-assessment is vital for nurses caring for clients who have personality disorders because of the intense emotions that can be elicited during client care.

    B. Underlying Principles
    - Self-assessment prepares the nurse for the personal emotions that can be experienced as a result of client care.
    - The nurse can provide more effective nursing care when aware of personal reactions to stress.
    - Therapeutic communication and intervention are promoted when client behaviors are anticipated.

    C. Nursing Interventions
    - Who: Self-assessment should be performed by all nurses caring for a client who has a personality disorder.
    - When: The nurse should perform a self-assessment prior to providing client care and whenever experiencing a personal stress response to client behavior.

    Ⓝ NCLEX® Connection: Psychosocial Integrity, Mental Health Concepts

UNIT 3   PSYCHOBIOLOGIC DISORDERS

CHAPTER 16   Cognitive Disorders

Overview

- Cognitive disorders are a group of conditions characterized by the disruption of thinking, memory, processing, and problem-solving.
- Treatment of clients who have cognitive disorders requires a compassionate understanding of both the client and the family.
- The various cognitive disorders recognized and defined by the DSM-5 include the following categories.
  - Delirium
  - Neurocognitive Disorder (can be classified as mild or major)
    - Alzheimer's disease is a subtype of neurocognitive disorder that is neurodegenerative, resulting in the gradual impairment of cognitive function.
- It is important to distinguish between a cognitive disorder and other mental health disorders that can have similar manifestations. Depression in the older adult can mimic the early stages of Alzheimer's disease.

Data Collection

- Risk Factors
  - Risk factors for delirium include physiological changes.
    - Neurological diseases (Parkinson's disease, Huntington's disease)
    - Metabolic diseases (hepatic or renal failure, fluid and electrolyte imbalances, nutritional deficiencies)
    - Cardiovascular diseases
    - Infections (HIV/AIDS)
    - Substance use or withdrawal
    - Most common in older adult clients and clients in an intensive care unit
  - Risk factors for neurocognitive disorder and Alzheimer's disease include a disorder of the neurological system, advanced age, prior head trauma, genetic factors, and a family history of Alzheimer's disease and/or trisomy 21 (Down syndrome).

- Subjective and Objective Data
  - Delirium and neurocognitive disorder have some similarities and some important differences.

DELIRIUM	NEUROCOGNITIVE DISORDER
Onset	
› Rapid over a short period of time (hours or days)	› Gradual deterioration of function over months or years
Clinical Manifestations	
› Occurrence of impairments in memory, judgment, ability to focus, and ability to calculate. These impairments can fluctuate throughout the day. › Level of consciousness is usually altered and can rapidly fluctuate. › Restlessness, agitation, and fluctuating mood are common. Sundowning (confusion during the night) can occur. Behaviors can increase or decrease daily. › Personality change is rapid. › Some perceptual disturbances, such as hallucinations and illusions, can be present. › Vital signs can be unstable and abnormal due to medical illness.	› Impairments in memory, judgment, speech (aphasia), ability to recognize familiar objects (agnosia), executive functioning (managing daily tasks), and movement (apraxia) do not change throughout the day. › Level of consciousness is usually unchanged. › Restlessness, agitation are common. Sundowning can occur. Behaviors usually remain stable. › Personality change is gradual. › Vital signs are stable unless other illness is present.
Cause	

› Caused secondary to another medical condition, such as infection, or to substance use.	› Cognitive deficits are not related to another mental health disorder.
	› Subtypes of neurocognitive disorder can be related to:
	  » Alzheimer's disease.
	  » Traumatic brain injury.
	  » Parkinson's disease.
	  » Other disorders affecting the neurological system.

Outcome	
› Reversible if diagnosis and treatment are prompt	› Irreversible and progressive

STAGES OF ALZHEIMER'S DISEASE: CLINICAL MANIFESTATIONS

Stage 1: No impairment (normal function)

› No memory problems	› No memory problems evident to provider

Stage 2: Very mild cognitive decline, which can be normal age-related changes or very early signs of Alzheimer's disease

› Forgetfulness, especially of everyday objects (eyeglasses, wallet)	› No memory problems evident to provider, friends, or coworkers

Stage 3: Mild cognitive decline, including problems with memory or concentration that can be measurable in clinical testing or during a detailed medical interview

› Mild cognitive deficits, including losing or misplacing important objects, decreased ability to plan › Short-term memory loss noticeable to close relations	› Decreased attention span › Difficulty remembering words or names › Difficulty in social or work situations

Stage 4: Moderate cognitive decline (mild or early-stage Alzheimer's disease) that is clearly detected during a medical interview

› Personality change: appearing withdrawn or subdued, especially in social or mentally challenging situations › Obvious memory loss	› Limited knowledge and memory of recent occasions, current events, or personal history › Difficulty performing tasks that require planning and organizing (paying bills, managing money) › Difficulty with complex mental arithmetic

Stage 5: Moderately severe cognitive decline (moderate or mid-stage Alzheimer's disease)

› Increasing cognitive deficits › Disorientation and confusion as to time and place	› Inability to recall important details, such as address and telephone number, but ability to remember information about self and family

Stage 6: Severe cognitive decline (moderately severe or mid-stage Alzheimer's disease)

› Continued worsening of memory difficulties › Loss of awareness of recent events and surroundings › Ability to recall own name but not personal history › Evidence of significant personality changes (delusions, hallucinations, compulsive behaviors) › Wandering behavior	› Assistance required for usual daily activities, such as dressing, toileting, and other grooming › Disruption of normal sleep/wake cycle › Increased episodes of urinary and fecal incontinence › Violent tendencies with potential danger to self or others

Stage 7: Very severe cognitive decline (severe or late-stage Alzheimer's disease)

› Loss of ability to respond to environment, to speak, and to control movement › Unrecognizable speech, general urinary incontinence, inability to eat without assistance, and impaired swallowing	› Gradual loss of all ability to move › Stupor and coma › Death frequently related to choking or infection

Retrieved 10.12.12 from www.alz.org

- Defense Mechanisms Used in Cognitive Disorders

  - Monitor for defense mechanisms used by the client to preserve self-esteem and to compensate when cognitive changes are progressive.

    - Denial – Both the client and family members can refuse to believe that changes, such as loss of memory, are taking place, even when those changes are obvious to others.

    - Confabulation – The client can make up stories when questioned about events or activities that she does not remember. This can seem like lying, but it is actually an unconscious attempt to save self-esteem and prevent admitting that she does not remember the occasion.

    - Perseveration – The client avoids answering questions by repeating phrases or behavior. This is another unconscious attempt to maintain self-esteem when memory has failed.

- Laboratory and Diagnostic Tests

  - Chest and skull x-rays

  - Electroencephalography (EEG)

  - Electrocardiography (ECG)

  - Liver function studies

  - Thyroid function tests

  - Neuroimaging (computer tomography and position emission tomography of the brain)

  - Urinalysis

  - Serum electrolytes

- Standardized Screening Tools

  - Functional Dementia Scale

    - Use of this tool will give the nurse information regarding the client's ability to perform self-care, the extent of the client's memory loss, mood changes, and the degree of danger to self and/or others.

  - Mental or Mini-Mental State Examination

  - Functional Assessment Screening Tool

  - Global Deterioration Scale

  - Blessed Dementia Scale

    - This tool provides the nurse with client behavioral information based on an interview with a secondary source such as a client's family member.

Patient-Centered Care

- Nursing Care
  - Perform self-assessment regarding possible feelings of frustration, anger, or fear when performing daily care for clients who have progressive cognitive decline.
  - Nursing interventions are focused on protecting the client from injury, as well as promoting client dignity and quality of life.

  - Provide for a safe and therapeutic environment
    - Assign the client to a room close to the nurses' station for close observation.
    - Provide a room with a low level of visual and auditory stimuli.
    - Provide for a well-lit environment, minimizing contrasts and shadows.
    - Have the client sit in a room with windows to help with time orientation.
    - Have the client wear an identification bracelet. Use monitors and bed alarm devices as needed.
    - Use restraints only as an intervention of last resort.
    - Monitor the client's level of comfort for non-verbal indications of discomfort.
    - Use caution when administering medications PRN for agitation or anxiety.
    - Check the client's risk for injury and ensure safety in the physical environment, such as a lowered bed and removal of scatter rugs to prevent falls.
    - Provide compensatory memory aids, such as clocks, calendars, photographs, memorabilia, seasonal decorations, and familiar objects. Reorient as necessary.
    - Provide eyeglasses and assistive hearing devices as needed.
    - Keep a consistent daily routine.
    - Maintain consistent caregivers.
    - Ensure adequate food and fluid intake.
    - Allow for safe pacing and wandering.
    - Cover or remove mirrors to decrease fear and agitation.
  - Communication
    - Communicate in a calm, reassuring tone.
    - Speak in positive rather than negatively worded phrases. Do not argue or question hallucinations or delusions.
    - Reinforce reality.
    - Reinforce orientation to time, place, and person.
    - Introduce self to client with each new contact.
    - Establish eye contact and use short, simple sentences when speaking to the client. Focus on one item of information at a time.
    - Encourage reminiscence about happy times. Talk about familiar things.
    - Break instructions and activities into short time frames.

- Limit the number of choices when dressing or eating.

- Minimize the need for decision-making and abstract thinking to avoid frustration.

- Avoid confrontation.

- Encourage family visitation as appropriate.

- Medications

  ○ Delirium

    - Pharmacological management focuses on the treatment of the underlying disorder. Antipsychotic or antianxiety medications can be prescribed.

  ○ Neurocognitive Disorder

    - Medications such as donepezil (Aricept), rivastigmine (Exelon), and galantamine (Razadyne) increase acetylcholine at cholinergic synapses by inhibiting its breakdown by acetylcholinesterase, which increases the availability of acetylcholine at neurotransmitter receptor sites in the CNS.

    - Therapeutic uses of these medications include improved ability to perform self-care and slow cognitive deterioration of Alzheimer's disease for clients in the mild to moderate stages.

MEDICATIONS FOR NEUROCOGNITIVE DISORDER

Adverse Effects	Nursing Interventions/Client Education
› Nausea and diarrhea, which occur in approximately 10% of clients	› Monitor for gastrointestinal adverse effects and fluid volume deficits. › Promote adequate fluid intake. › The provider can titrate the dosage to reduce gastrointestinal effects.
› Bradycardia	› Instruct the client's family to monitor pulse rate for the client who lives at home. › The client should be screened for underlying heart disease.

    - Contraindications/precautions

      □ The cholinesterase inhibitors should be used with caution in clients who have pre-existing asthma or other obstructive pulmonary disorders. Bronchoconstriction can be caused by an increase of acetylcholine.

MEDICATION CONTRAINDICATIONS/PRECAUTIONS

Medication/Food Interactions	Nursing Interventions/Client Education
› Concurrent use of NSAIDs, such as aspirin, can cause gastrointestinal bleeding.	› Check the use of over-the-counter NSAIDs. › Monitor for indications of gastrointestinal bleeding.
› Antihistamines, tricyclic antidepressants, and conventional antipsychotics (medications that block cholinergic receptors) can reduce the therapeutic effects of donepezil.	› Use of cholinergic receptor blocking medications for clients taking any cholinesterase inhibitor is not recommended.

- Nursing considerations
  - Dosage should start low and gradually be increased until adverse effects are no longer tolerable or medication is no longer beneficial.
  - Monitor for adverse effects, and inform the client and family about these effects. Taper medication when discontinuing to prevent abrupt progression of clinical manifestations.
  - Monitor the client for the ability to swallow tablets. Most of the medications are available in tablets and oral solutions. Donepezil is available in an orally disintegrating tablet.
  - Administer with or without food.
  - Donepezil has a long half-life and is administered once daily at bedtime. The other cholinesterase inhibitors usually are administered twice daily.
- Medications such as memantine (Namenda) block the entry of calcium into nerve cells, thus slowing down brain-cell death.
  - Memantine is the only medication approved for moderate to severe stages of Alzheimer's disease.
  - Nursing considerations
    - Memantine can be used concurrently with a cholinesterase inhibitor.
    - Administer the medication with or without food.
    - Monitor for common adverse effects, including dizziness, headache, confusion, and constipation.

- Alternative/Complementary Therapies
  - Estrogen therapy for women can prevent Alzheimer's disease, but it is not useful in decreasing the effects of pre-existing cognitive deficits.
  - Ginkgo biloba, an herbal product, is used by some clients to enhance memory. Tell clients to inform the provider of the use of ginkgo biloba due to potential interactions, such as the risk for bleeding in clients taking antiplatelet medications, as well as the risk for seizures in clients taking medications that can lower seizure threshold.

- Care After Discharge
  - Reinforce teaching to family/caregivers about the client's illness, methods of care, and adaptation of the home environment.

  - Ensure a safe environment in the home. Questions to ask include:
    - Will the client wander out into the street if doors are left unlocked?
    - Is the client able to remember his address and his name?
    - Does the client harm others when allowed to wander in a long-term care facility?

- Home safety measures to be implemented can include the following.
    - Removing scatter rugs
    - Installing door locks that cannot be easily opened
    - Locking water heater thermostat and turning water temperature down to a safe level
    - Providing good lighting, especially on stairs
    - Installing a handrail on stairs, and marking step edges with colored tape
    - Placing mattresses on the floor
    - Removing clutter, keeping clear, wide pathways for walking through a room
    - Securing electrical cords to baseboards
    - Storing cleaning supplies in locked cupboards
    - Installing handrails in bathrooms
  - Monitor for improvement in memory and the client's quality of life.
- Support for Caregivers

  - Determine teaching needs for the client and especially the client's family members as cognitive ability progressively declines.
  - Review the resources available to the family as the client's health declines. Include long-term care options. A wide variety of home care and community resources can be available to the family in many areas of the country. These resources can allow the client to remain at home, rather than in a care facility.
  - Provide support for caregivers. Recommend local support groups for caregivers, as well as respite care.
  - Establish a routine. Make sure all caregivers know and apply the routine. Attempt to have consistency in caregivers.

APPLICATION EXERCISES

1. A nurse is caring for a client who has Alzheimer's disease and is beginning to experience noticeable short-term memory loss. When discussing a new prescription for donepezil (Aricept), the nurse should include which of the following in the instructions?

    A. "You should avoid taking over-the-counter acetaminophen while on donepezil."

    B. "You can expect the progression of cognitive decline to slow with donepezil."

    C. "You will be screened for underlying kidney disease prior to starting donepezil."

    D. "You should stop taking donepezil if you experience nausea or diarrhea."

2. A nurse in a long-term care facility is caring for a resident who has major neurocognitive disorder and attempts to wander out of the building. The client states, "I have to get home." Which of the following is an appropriate response by the nurse?

    A. "You have forgotten that this is your home."

    B. "You cannot go outside without a staff member."

    C. "Why would you want to leave? Aren't you happy with your care?"

    D. "I am your nurse. Let's walk together to your room."

3. A nurse is making a home visit to a client who has Alzheimer's disease to collect data regarding home safety. Which of the following are appropriate suggestions to decrease the client's risk for injury?

    _____ A. Install childproof door locks.

    _____ B. Place rugs over electrical cords.

    _____ C. Mark cleaning supplies with colored tape.

    _____ D. Place the client's mattress on the floor.

    _____ E. Install light fixtures above stairs.

4. A nurse is making a home visit to a client who is in the late stage of Alzheimer's disease. The client's spouse, who is the primary caregiver, wishes to discuss concerns about the client's nutrition and the stress of providing care. Which of the following is an appropriate action by the nurse?

    A. Verify that a current power of attorney document is on file.

    B. Tell the client's spouse to offer finger foods to increase oral intake.

    C. Provide information on resources for respite care.

    D. Schedule the client for placement of an enteral feeding tube.

5. A nurse is assisting with data collection for a client who has delirium related to an acute urinary tract infection. Which of the following are expected findings? (Select all that apply.)

_____ A. History of gradual memory loss

_____ B. Family report of personality changes

_____ C. Hallucinations

_____ D. Unaltered level of consciousness

_____ E. Restlessness

6. A nurse is assisting with planning care to promote a safe and therapeutic environment for a client who has severe cognitive decline due to Alzheimer's disease. Use the ATI Active Learning Template: Systems Disorder to complete this item to include the following:

A. Description of Disorder/Disease Process

B. Collaborative Care: Nursing Care – Identify five nursing actions.

APPLICATION EXERCISES KEY

1. A. INCORRECT: Clients taking donepezil should avoid NSAIDs, rather than acetaminophen, due to risk for gastrointestinal bleeding.

   B. **CORRECT:** Donepezil slows the cognitive deterioration of Alzheimer's disease.

   C. INCORRECT: Clients should be screened for underlying heart and pulmonary disease, rather than kidney disease, prior to treatment.

   D. INCORRECT: Gastrointestinal adverse effects are common with donepezil and can result in a dosage reduction. However, the client should not abruptly stop the medication without consulting his provider.

   Ⓝ NCLEX® Connection: Basic Care and Comfort, Mobility/Immobility

2. A. INCORRECT: The nurse should avoid statements that can be interpreted as argumentative or demeaning.

   B. INCORRECT: The nurse should use positive rather than negative statements.

   C. INCORRECT: Using a "why" question can promote a defensive reaction and does not reinforce reality.

   D. **CORRECT:** It is appropriate for the nurse to introduce herself with each new interaction and to promote reality in a calm, reassuring manner.

   Ⓝ NCLEX® Connection: Psychosocial Integrity, Mental Health Concepts

3. A. **CORRECT:** Door locks that are difficult to open are appropriate to reduce the risk of the client wandering outside without supervision.

   B. INCORRECT: Rugs create a fall risk hazard and should be removed. Electrical cords should be secured to baseboards rather than covered.

   C. INCORRECT: Cleaning supplies should be placed in locked cupboards. Marking the supplies with colored tape does not prevent the client's access to hazardous materials.

   D. **CORRECT:** Placing the client's mattress on the floor reduces the risk for falls out of bed.

   E. **CORRECT:** Stairs should have adequate lighting to reduce the risk for falls.

   Ⓝ NCLEX® Connection: Psychosocial Integrity, Mental Health Concepts

4. A. INCORRECT: A power of attorney document does not address the client's care or the concerns of the caregiver.

   B. INCORRECT: Clients in late-stage Alzheimer's disease are at risk for choking and are unable to eat without assistance. Therefore, offering finger foods is not an appropriate action.

   C. **CORRECT:** Providing information on resources for respite care is an appropriate action to provide the client's spouse with a break from caregiving responsibilities.

   D. INCORRECT: Placement of an enteral feeding tube is appropriate only with a prescription from the provider following a discussion that includes the provider, nurse, the client's spouse, as well as possibly social services and additional family members.

   Ⓝ NCLEX® Connection: Coordinated Care, Referral Process

5. A. INCORRECT: The client who has delirium can experience memory loss with sudden rather than gradual onset.

    B. **CORRECT:** The client who has delirium can experience rapid personality changes.

    C. **CORRECT:** The client who has delirium can have perceptual disturbances, such as hallucinations and illusions.

    D. INCORRECT: The client who has delirium is expected to have an altered level of consciousness that can rapidly fluctuate.

    E. **CORRECT:** The client who has delirium commonly exhibits restlessness and agitation.

    Ⓝ NCLEX® Connection: Physiological Adaptations, Basic Pathophysiology

6. *Using the ATI Active Learning Template: Systems Disorder*

    A. Description of Disorder/Disease Process

    • Alzheimer's disease is a subtype of neurocognitive disorder that is neurodegenerative, resulting in the gradual impairment of cognitive function. A client who has severe cognitive decline has memory difficulties, loss of awareness to recent events and surroundings, inability to recall personal history, personality changes, wandering behavior, the need for assistance with ADLs, disruption of sleep/wake cycle, and violent tendencies.

    B. Collaborative Care: Nursing Care

    • Assign a room close to the nurses' station.

    • Provide a room with a low level of visual and auditory stimuli.

    • Provide for a well-lit environment, minimizing contrasts and shadows.

    • Have the client sit in a room with windows to help with time orientation.

    • Have the client wear an identification bracelet. Use monitors and bed alarm devices as needed.

    • Monitor the client's level of comfort.

    • Provide compensatory memory aids, such as clocks, calendars, photographs, memorabilia, seasonal decorations, and familiar objects. Reorient as necessary.

    • Provide eyeglasses and assistive hearing devices as needed.

    • Keep a consistent daily routine.

    • Maintain consistent caregivers.

    • Ensure adequate food and fluid intake.

    • Allow for safe pacing and wandering.

    • Cover or remove mirrors to decrease fear and agitation.

    Ⓝ NCLEX® Connection: Psychosocial Integrity, Mental Health Concepts

UNIT 3   PSYCHOBIOLOGIC DISORDERS

CHAPTER 17   Substance Use and Addictive Disorders

Overview

- Substance use and addictive disorders recognized and defined by the DSM-5 include the following.
  - Substance use disorders are related to alcohol, cannabis, hallucinogens, inhalants, opioids, sedatives/hypnotics, stimulants, and tobacco.
  - A substance use disorder involves a repeated use of chemical substances, leading to clinically significant impairment during a 12-month period, and at least two of the following criteria.
    - Uses substance in larger amounts or over a longer period of time than intended.
    - Has a continued desire or unsuccessful attempt to control substance use.
    - Spends a considerable amount of time obtaining, using, or recovering from the effects of the substance.
    - Continues to use the substance regardless of social or interpersonal problems associated with substance use.
    - Reduces or quits participation in social, occupational, or recreational activities because of substance use.
    - Uses the substance repeatedly in physically hazardous situations, such as driving impaired.
    - Continues to use the substance regardless of physical or psychological problems associated with substance use.
    - Develops a tolerance to the substance.
    - Requires additional amounts of the substance to achieve the desired effect or to become intoxicated.
    - Exhibits manifestations of withdrawal.
    - Feels a strong urge to use the substance.
  - Severity scale for substance use disorder.
    - 0 or 1 criteria = no diagnosis of substance use disorder
    - 2 or 3 criteria = mild substance use disorder
    - 4 or 5 criteria = moderate substance use disorder
    - 6 or more criteria = severe substance use disorder

- Non-substance-related disorders (process addictions) include problematic behavior related to the following examples.

  - Gambling

  - Sexual behaviors

  - Shopping/spending

  - Internet use, such as gaming

- Addiction is characterized by:

  - Loss of control due to addictive behavior.

  - Participation that continues despite continuing associated problems.

  - A tendency to relapse back into the addictive behavior.

- The defense mechanism of denial is commonly used by clients who have problems with substance use or an addictive disorder. For example, a person who has long-term tobacco use might say, "I can quit whenever I want to, but smoking really doesn't cause me any problems." Denial often prevents a client from obtaining help with substance use or an addictive behavior.

Data Collection

- Risk Factors

  - Genetics – Predisposition to developing a substance use disorder due to family history

  - Lowered self-esteem

  - Lowered tolerance for pain and frustration

  - Few meaningful personal relationships

  - Few life successes

  - Risk-taking tendencies

  - Sociocultural theories

    - Certain cultures within the United States, such as Native American groups, have a high percentage of members who have alcohol use disorder. Other cultures, such as Asian groups, have a low percentage of alcohol use disorder.

      - Metabolism of alcohol and cultural views of alcohol use provide possible explanations for the incidence of alcohol use within a cultural group.

    - Peer pressure and other sociologic factors can increase the likelihood of substance use.

   - The older adult client can have a history of alcohol use or can develop a pattern of alcohol/substance use later in life due to life stressors, such as losing a spouse or a friend, retirement, or social isolation.

- Subjective and Objective Data
  - The nurse should use open-ended questions to obtain the following information for the nursing history.
    - Type of substance or addictive behavior
    - Pattern and frequency of substance use
    - Amount of substance used
    - Age at onset of substance use
    - Changes in occupational or school performance
    - Changes in use patterns
    - Periods of abstinence in history
    - Previous withdrawal manifestations
    - Date of last substance use or addictive behavior
    - Review of systems
      - Blackout or loss of consciousness
      - Changes in bowel movements
      - Weight loss or gain
      - Experience of stressful situation
      - Sleep problems
      - Chronic pain
      - Concern over substance use
      - Cutting down on consumption or behavior
  - Considerations for Specific Populations
    - Approximately half of college students participate in binge drinking or substance use every month.
    - The percentage of college students who use alcohol or have alcohol use disorder is significantly higher than the general population.
    - Anabolic steroid use is a growing concern among adolescents and young adults, especially athletes. The substance, known by names such as juice, gym candy, or stackers, can be taken orally or by injection in an attempt to improve physical appearance or performance. Negative effects include possible liver damage, hypertension, and infertility.

    - Older adults who use substances are especially prone to falls and other injuries, memory loss, somatic reports (headaches), and changes in sleep patterns.
      - Indications of alcohol use in the older adult can include a decrease in ability for self-care (functional status), urinary incontinence, and signs of dementia.
      - Older adults can show effects of alcohol use at lower doses than younger adults.
      - Polypharmacy (the use of multiple medications), the potential interaction between substances and medication, and age-related physiological changes raise the likelihood of adverse effects, such as confusion and falls, in older adult clients.

- Central Nervous System Depressants
  - CNS depressants can produce physiological and psychological dependence and can have cross-tolerance, cross-dependency, and an additive effect when take concurrently.

CENTRAL NERVOUS SYSTEM DEPRESSANTS	
ALCOHOL (ETHANOL)	
General Information	› A laboratory blood alcohol concentration (BAC) of 0.08% (80 g/dL) is considered legally intoxicated for adults operating automobiles in every U.S. state. Death can occur from acute toxicity in levels greater than 0.35% (350 g/dL).
	› BAC depends on many factors, including body weight, gender, concentration of alcohol in drinks, number of drinks, gastric absorption rate, and the individual's tolerance level.
Intended Effects	› Relaxation, decreased social anxiety, stress reduction
Effects of Intoxication	› Effects of excess – slurred speech, nystagmus, memory impairment, altered judgment, decreased motor skills, decreased level of consciousness (which can include stupor or coma), respiratory arrest, peripheral collapse, and death (with large doses)
	› Chronic use – direct cardiovascular damage, liver damage (ranging from fatty liver to cirrhosis), erosive gastritis and gastrointestinal bleeding, acute pancreatitis, sexual dysfunction
Withdrawal Manifestations	› Effects usually start within 4 to 12 hr of the last intake of alcohol, peak after 24 to 48 hr, and then suddenly disappear.
	› Manifestations include abdominal cramping; vomiting; tremors; restlessness and inability to sleep; increased heart rate; transient hallucinations or illusions; anxiety; increased blood pressure, respiratory rate, and temperature; and tonic-clonic seizures.
	› Alcohol withdrawal delirium can occur 2 to 3 days after cessation of alcohol and can last 2 to 3 days. This is considered a medical emergency. Clinical findings include severe disorientation, psychotic symptoms (hallucinations), severe hypertension, cardiac dysrhythmias, and delirium. Clinical findings can progress to death.
SEDATIVES/HYPNOTICS	
General Information	› Benzodiazepines like diazepam (Valium) or barbiturates like pentobarbital (Nembutal Sodium) can be taken orally or injected.
Intended Effects	› Decreased anxiety, sedation
Effects of Intoxication	› Increased drowsiness and sedation, agitation, slurred speech, uncoordinated motor activity, nystagmus, disorientation, nausea, vomiting
	› Respiratory depression and decreased level of consciousness, which can be fatal
	› An antidote, flumazenil, can be used IV for benzodiazepine toxicity
	› No antidote to reverse barbiturate toxicity
Withdrawal Manifestations	› Anxiety, insomnia, diaphoresis, hypertension, possible psychotic reactions, hand tremors, nausea or vomiting, hallucinations or illusions, psychomotor agitation, and sometimes seizure activity

CANNABIS	
General Information	› Marijuana or hashish (which is more potent) can be smoked or orally ingested.
Intended Effects	› Euphoria, sedation, hallucinations, decrease of nausea and vomiting secondary to chemotherapy, management of chronic pain
Effects of Intoxication	› Chronic use – lung cancer, chronic bronchitis, and other respiratory effects › In high doses, occurrence of paranoia, such as delusions and hallucinations › Increased appetite, dry mouth, tachycardia
Withdrawal Manifestations	› Irritability, aggression, anxiety, insomnia, lack of appetite, restlessness, depressed mood, abdominal pain, tremors, diaphoresis, fever, headache

- Central Nervous System Stimulants
  - The CNS stimulation seen in specific CNS stimulants is dependent on the area of the brain and spinal cord affected.

CENTRAL NERVOUS SYSTEM STIMULANTS	
COCAINE	
General Information	› Can be injected, smoked, or inhaled (snorted)
Intended Effects	› Rush of euphoria and pleasure, increased energy
Effects of Intoxication	› Mild toxicity – dizziness, irritability, tremor, blurred vision › Severe effects – hallucinations, seizures, extreme fever, tachycardia, hypertension, chest pain, cardiovascular collapse, death
Withdrawal Manifestations	› Characteristic withdrawal syndrome occurring within 1 hr to several days of cessation of drug use › Depression, fatigue, craving, excess sleeping or insomnia, dramatic unpleasant dreams, psychomotor retardation or agitation › Not life-threatening, but possible occurrence of suicidal ideation
AMPHETAMINES	
General Information	› Can be taken orally, injected intravenously, or smoked
Intended Effects	› Increased energy, euphoria similar to cocaine
Effects of Intoxication	› Impaired judgment, psychomotor agitation, hypervigilance, extreme irritability › Acute cardiovascular effects (tachycardia, elevated blood pressure), which can cause death
Withdrawal Manifestations	› Craving, depression, fatigue, sleeping (similar to those of cocaine) › Not life-threatening

CENTRAL NERVOUS SYSTEM STIMULANTS

TOBACCO (NICOTINE)

General Information	› Cigarettes and cigars are inhaled; smokeless tobacco is snuffed or chewed.
Intended Effects	› Relaxation, decreased anxiety
Effects of Intoxication	› Highly toxic, but acute toxicity seen only in children or when exposure is to nicotine in pesticides › Contains other harmful chemicals that are highly toxic and have long-term effects › Long-term effects – cardiovascular disease (hypertension, stroke); respiratory disease (emphysema, lung cancer); irritation to oral mucous membranes and cancer with smokeless tobacco (snuff or "chew")
Withdrawal Manifestations	› Abstinence syndrome is evidenced by irritability, craving, nervousness, restlessness, anxiety, insomnia, increased appetite, difficulty concentrating, anger, and depressed mood.

OPIOIDS

General Information	› Heroin, morphine, and hydromorphone (Dilaudid) can be injected, smoked, and inhaled.
Intended Effects	› A rush of euphoria (extreme well-being), relief from pain
Effects of Intoxication	› Slurred speech, impaired memory, pupillary changes, and decreased respirations and level of consciousness, which can cause death › Maladaptive behavioral or psychological changes, including impaired judgment or social functioning › An antidote, naloxone (Narcan), available for IV use to relieve effects of overdose
Withdrawal Manifestations	› Abstinence syndrome begins with sweating and rhinorrhea progressing to piloerection (gooseflesh), tremors, and irritability followed by severe weakness, diarrhea, fever, insomnia, pupil dilation, nausea and vomiting, pain in the muscles and bones, and muscle spasms. › Withdrawal is very unpleasant but not life-threatening, and it is self-limiting to 7 to 10 days.

INHALANTS

General Information	› Amyl nitrate, nitrous oxide, and solvents are "sniffed," "huffed," or "bagged," often by children or teenagers.
Intended Effects	› Euphoria
Effects of Intoxication	› Depending on the substance, behavioral or psychological changes, dizziness, nystagmus, uncoordinated movements or gait, slurred speech, drowsiness, hyporeflexia, muscle weakness, diplopia, stupor or coma, respiratory depression, death
Withdrawal Manifestations	› None

HALLUCINOGENS	
General Information	› Lysergic acid diethylamide (LSD), mescaline (peyote), and phencyclidine piperidine (PCP) are usually ingested orally, can be injected or smoked
Intended Effects	› Heightened sense of self and altered perceptions (colors being more vivid while under the influence)
Effects of Intoxication	› Anxiety, depression, paranoia, impaired judgment and social functioning, pupil dilation, tachycardia, diaphoresis, palpitations, blurred vision, tremors, incoordination, and panic attacks
Withdrawal Manifestations	› Hallucinogen persisting perception disorder – Visual disturbances or flashback hallucinations can occur intermittently for years.

- Designer or club drugs, such as ecstasy, can combine substances from different categories, producing varying effects of intoxication or withdrawal.

- Improper use of prescription medications, specifically opioids, CNS depressants, and CNS stimulants, can result in substance use disorder and drug-seeking behavior.

- Standardized Screening Tools

  - Michigan Alcohol Screening Test (MAST) or Michigan Alcohol Screening Test – Geriatric (MAST-G)
  - Addiction Severity Index
  - Recovery Attitude and Treatment Evaluator
  - Drug Abuse Screening Test (DAST)
  - CAGE-AID asks questions of clients to determine how clients perceive their current substance use.

Patient-Centered Care

- Nursing Care

  - Personal views, culture, and history can affect the nurse's feelings regarding substance use and addictive disorders. The nurse must self-assess his own feelings, which can be transferred to the client through body language and the terminology the nurse uses when collecting data from the client. An objective, nonjudgmental approach by the nurse is imperative.

  - Safety is the primary focus of nursing care during acute intoxication or withdrawal.

    - Maintain a safe environment to prevent falls. Implement seizure precautions as necessary.
    - Provide close observation for withdrawal symptoms, possibly one-on-one supervision. Physical restraint should be a last resort.
    - Orient the client to time, place, and person.
    - Maintain adequate nutrition and fluid balance.
    - Create a low-stimulation environment.
    - Administer medications to treat the effects of intoxication or to prevent or manage withdrawal.
    - Monitor for covert substance use during the detoxification period.

- ○ Provide emotional support and reassurance to the client and family.

- ○ Reinforce client and family education regarding codependent behaviors.

- ○ Reinforce client and family education about addiction and the initial treatment goal of abstinence.

- ○ Reinforce client and family education regarding removing any prescription medications in the home that are not being used. Encourage the client not to share medication with someone for whom that medication is not prescribed.

- ○ Begin to develop motivation and commitment for abstinence and recovery (abstinence plus working a program of personal growth and self-discovery).

- ○ Encourage self-responsibility.

- ○ Help the client develop an emergency plan – a list of things the client would need to do and people he would need to contact.

- ○ Encourage attendance at self-help groups.

- Teamwork and Collaboration

  - ○ Dual diagnosis, or comorbidity, means that an individual has both a mental illness, such as depression, as well as a problem with substance use or an addictive disorder. Both disorders need to be treated simultaneously and will require a team approach.

  - ○ Individual psychotherapies

    - Cognitive behavioral therapies, such as relaxation techniques or cognitive reframing, can be used to decrease anxiety and change behavior.

    - Acceptance and commitment therapy (ACT) promotes acceptance of the client's experiences and promotes client commitment to positive behavior changes.

    - Relapse prevention therapy (RPT) assists clients in identifying the potential for relapse and promotes behavioral self-control.

  - ○ Group therapy

    - Groups of clients who have similar diagnoses can meet in an outpatient setting or within mental health residential facilities.

  - ○ Family therapy

    - This therapy identifies codependency, which is a common behavior demonstrated by the significant other, family, and friends of an individual who has substance or process dependency, and assists the family to change that behavior. The codependent person reacts in over-responsible ways that allow the dependent individual to continue the substance use or addiction disorder. For example, a spouse can act as an enabler by calling the client's employer with an excuse of illness when the client is intoxicated.

    - Families learn about use of specific substances.

    - The client and family are educated regarding such issues as family coping, problem solving, relapse signs, and availability of support groups.

- Pharmacological therapy
  - Medications
    - Alcohol withdrawal – diazepam (Valium), lorazepam (Ativan), carbamazepine (Tegretol), clonidine (Catapres), chlordiazepoxide (Librium)
    - Alcohol abstinence – disulfiram (Antabuse), naltrexone (Revia), acamprosate (Campral)
    - Opioid withdrawal – methadone (Dolophine) substitution, clonidine (Catapres), buprenorphine (Subutex)
    - Nicotine withdrawal from tobacco use – bupropion (Zyban), nicotine replacement therapy (nicotine gum [Nicorette] and nicotine patch [Nicotrol])
  - Nursing Considerations

    - Monitor and document vital signs and neurological status.
    - Provide for client safety by implementing seizure precautions.
  - Client Education
    - Encourage the client to adhere to the treatment plan.
    - Advise the client taking disulfiram to avoid all alcohol.
- Care After Discharge
  - Client Education
    - Reinforce the need to recognize indications of relapse and factors that contribute to relapse.
    - Reinforce cognitive-behavioral techniques to help maintain sobriety and to create feelings of pleasure from activities other than using substances or from process addictions.
    - Assist the client to develop communication skills to communicate with coworkers and family members while sober.
    - Encourage the client and family to attend a 12-step program, such as Alcoholics Anonymous (AA), Narcotics Anonymous, Gambler's Anonymous, and family groups like Al-Anon or Ala-Teen.
      - These programs will teach clients the following.
        - Abstinence is necessary for recovery.
        - A higher power is needed to assist in recovery.
        - Clients are not responsible for their disease but are responsible for their recovery.
        - Others cannot be blamed for clients' addictions, and they must acknowledge their feelings and problems.

APPLICATION EXERCISES

1. A nurse is assisting with the preparation of a staff education program on substance use in older adults. Which of the following is appropriate for the nurse to include in the presentation?

    A. Older adults require higher doses of a substance to achieve a desired effect.

    B. Older adults commonly use rationalization to cope with a substance use disorder.

    C. Older adults are at a higher risk for substance use following retirement.

    D. Older adults develop substance use to mask signs of dementia.

2. A nurse is monitoring a client who has alcohol use disorder and is experiencing withdrawal. Which of the following is an expected finding? (Select all that apply.)

    _____ A. Bradycardia

    _____ B. Fine tremors of both hands

    _____ C. Hypotension

    _____ D. Vomiting

    _____ E. Restlessness

3. A nurse is assisting with planning care for a client who is experiencing benzodiazepine withdrawal. Which of the following is the priority nursing intervention?

    A. Orient the client frequently to time, place, and person.

    B. Offer fluids and nourishing diet as tolerated.

    C. Implement seizure precautions.

    D. Encourage participation in group therapy sessions.

4. A nurse is caring for a client who has alcohol use disorder. The client is no longer experiencing withdrawal manifestations. Which of the following medications should the nurse anticipate administering to assist the client with maintaining abstinence from alcohol?

    A. Chlordiazepoxide (Librium)

    B. Bupropion (Zyban)

    C. Disulfiram (Antabuse)

    D. Carbamazepine (Tegretol)

5. A nurse is reinforcing teaching to the family of a client who has a substance use disorder. Which of the following statements by a family member indicates a need for further teaching?

    A. "We need to understand that she is not responsible for her disorder."

    B. "Eliminating any codependent behavior will promote her recovery."

    C. "She should participate in an Al-Anon group to help her recover."

    D. "The primary goal of her treatment is abstinence from substance use."

6. A nurse is caring for a client who has moderate cocaine use disorder and is experiencing severe effects of intoxication. Use the ATI Active Learning Template: Systems Disorder to complete this item to include the following:

    A. Description of Disorder/Disease Process

    B. Data Collection: Objective and Subjective – Identify three expected findings.

    C. Patient-Centered Care: Nursing Care – Describe two nursing interventions.

    D. Patient-Centered Care: Teamwork and Collaboration – Describe two forms of nonpharmacological therapy.

APPLICATION EXERCISES KEY

1. A. INCORRECT: Requiring higher doses of a substance to achieve a desired effect is a result of the length and severity of substance use rather than age.

    B. INCORRECT: Denial, rather than rationalization, is a defense mechanism commonly used by substance users of all ages.

    C. **CORRECT:** Retirement and other life change stressors increase the risk for substance use in older adults, especially if there is a prior history of substance use.

    D. INCORRECT: Substance use in the older adult can result in signs of dementia.

    (N) NCLEX® Connection: Psychosocial Integrity, Chemical and Other Dependencies

2. A. INCORRECT: An expected finding of alcohol withdrawal is tachycardia rather than bradycardia.

    B. **CORRECT:** Fine tremors of both hands is an expected finding of alcohol withdrawal.

    C. INCORRECT: An expected finding of alcohol withdrawal is hypertension rather than hypotension.

    D. **CORRECT:** Vomiting is an expected finding of alcohol withdrawal.

    E. **CORRECT:** Restlessness is an expected finding of alcohol withdrawal.

    (N) NCLEX® Connection: Psychosocial Integrity, Chemical and Other Dependencies

3. A. INCORRECT: Reorienting the client is an appropriate intervention. However, it is not the priority.

    B. INCORRECT: Providing hydration and nourishment is an appropriate intervention. However, it is not the priority.

    C. **CORRECT:** The greatest risk to the client is injury. Therefore, implementing seizure precautions is the priority intervention.

    D. INCORRECT: Encouraging participation in therapy is an appropriate intervention. However, it is not the priority.

    (N) NCLEX® Connection: Psychosocial Integrity, Chemical and Other Dependencies

4. A. INCORRECT: Chlordiazepoxide (Librium) is indicated for acute alcohol withdrawal rather than to maintain abstinence from alcohol.

    B. INCORRECT: Bupropion (Zyban) is indicated for nicotine withdrawal rather than to maintain abstinence from alcohol.

    C. **CORRECT:** Disulfiram (Antabuse) is administered to help clients maintain abstinence from alcohol.

    D. INCORRECT: Carbamazepine (Tegretol) is indicated for acute alcohol withdrawal rather than to maintain abstinence from alcohol.

    (N) NCLEX® Connection: Pharmacological Therapies, Expected Actions/Outcomes

5.   A. INCORRECT: Clients are not responsible for their disease but are responsible for their recovery.

      B. INCORRECT: Families should be aware of codependent behavior, such as enabling, that can promote substance use rather than recovery.

      C. **CORRECT:** Al-Anon is a recovery group for the family of a client, rather than the client who has a substance use disorder.

      D. INCORRECT: Abstinence is the primary treatment goal for a client who has a substance use disorder.

    Ⓝ NCLEX® Connection: Psychosocial Integrity, Chemical and Other Dependencies

6.   *Using the ATI Active Learning Template: Systems Disorder*

    A. Description of Disorder/Disease Process
- Cocaine use disorder involves the repeated use of cocaine, leading to clinically significant impairment over a 12-month period. Moderate cocaine use disorder indicates the client currently meets four or five of the criteria indicated by the DSM-5.

    B. Data Collection: Objective and Subjective
- Objective: Seizures, extreme fever, tachycardia, hypertension
- Subjective: Hallucinations, chest pain

    C. Patient-Centered Care: Nursing Care
- Perform a nursing self-assessment.
- Maintain a safe environment.
- Implement seizure precautions.
- Orient the client to time, place, and person.
- Create a low-stimulation environment.
- Monitor vital signs and neurological status.

    D. Patient-Centered Care: Teamwork and Collaboration
- Cognitive behavioral therapies decrease anxiety and promote a change in behavior.
- Acceptance and commitment therapy promotes acceptance of the client and promotes a commitment to change.
- Relapse prevention therapy assists clients in identifying relapse and promotes self-control.
- Group therapy allows clients who have similar diagnoses to work together toward recovery.
- Family therapy allows the client and family members to work together toward recovery.
- Narcotics Anonymous provides a 12-step program to promote recovery and abstinence from future narcotic use.

    Ⓝ NCLEX® Connection: Psychosocial Integrity, Chemical and Other Dependencies

chapter **18**

Overview

- Eating disorders recognized and defined by the DSM-5 include the following.
  - Anorexia nervosa
    - Clients are preoccupied with food and the rituals of eating, along with a voluntary refusal to eat.
    - Clients exhibit a morbid fear of obesity and a refusal to maintain a minimally normal body weight (body weight is less than 85% of expected weight for the individual) in the absence of a physical cause.
    - This condition occurs most often in females from adolescence to young adulthood. The average age of onset in females is 12 to 18 years of age.
    - Two types
      - Restricting type – The individual drastically restricts food intake and does not binge or purge.
      - Binge-eating/purging type – The individual engages in binge eating or purging behaviors.
  - Bulimia nervosa
    - Clients recurrently eat large quantities of food over a short period of time (binge eating), which can be followed by inappropriate compensatory behaviors, such as self-induced vomiting (purging), to rid the body of the excess calories.
    - Most clients who have bulimia nervosa maintain a weight within a normal range or slightly higher.
    - Bulimia nervosa occurs most commonly in females. Onset generally occurs between 18 and 26 years of age.
    - Two types
      - Purging type – The client uses self-induced vomiting, laxatives, diuretics, and/or enemas to lose or maintain weight.
      - Nonpurging type – The client can also compensate for binge eating through other means, such as excessive exercise and the misuse of laxatives, diuretics, and/or enemas.
  - Binge-eating disorder
    - Clients recurrently eat large quantities of food over a short period of time without the use of compensatory behaviors associated with bulimia nervosa.
    - Binge-eating disorder affects men and women of all ages, but is most common in adults age 46 to 55.
    - The weight gain associated with binge-eating disorder increases the client's risk for other disorders, including type 2 diabetes mellitus, hypertension, and cancer.

- Mortality rate for eating disorders is high. Suicide is also a risk.

- Treatment modalities focus on normalizing eating patterns and addressing the issues raised by the illness.

- Comorbidities include depression, personality disorders, substance use disorder, and anxiety.

Data Collection

- Risk Factors

  ○ Family genetics – families who have a history of eating disorders

  ○ Biological – hypothalamic, neurotransmitter, hormonal, or biochemical imbalance, with disturbances of the serotonin neurotransmitter pathways seeming to be implicated

  ○ Interpersonal relationships – influenced by parental pressure and the need to succeed

  ○ Psychological influences – rigidity, ritualism; separation and individuation conflicts; feelings of ineffectiveness, helplessness, and depression; distorted body image; internal or external locus of control or self-identity; history of physical abuse

  ○ Environmental factors – media influence and pressure from society to have the "perfect body," culture of abundance

  ○ History of being a "picky" eater in childhood

  ○ Participation in athletics, especially at an elite level of competition or in a sport where lean body build is prized (bicycling) or where a specific weight is necessary (wrestling)

  ○ History of obesity

- Subjective and Objective Data

  ○ Nursing history should include the following.

    ▪ The client's perception of the issue

    ▪ Eating habits

    ▪ History of dieting

    ▪ Methods of weight control (restricting, purging, exercising)

    ▪ Value attached to a specific shape and weight

    ▪ Interpersonal and social functioning

    ▪ Difficulty with impulsivity, as well as compulsivity

    ▪ Family and interpersonal relationships (frequently troublesome and chaotic, reflecting a lack of nurturing)

OBJECTIVE DATA	FINDINGS
Mental status	› Cognitive distortions
	» Overgeneralizations – "Other girls don't like me because I'm fat."
	» "All-or-nothing" thinking – "If I eat any dessert, I'll gain 50 pounds."
	» Catastrophizing – "My life is over if I gain weight."
	» Personalization – "When I walk through the hospital hallway, I know everyone is looking at me."
	» Emotional reasoning – "I know I look bad because I feel bloated."
	› Client demonstrates high interest in preparing food, but not eating.
	› Client is terrified of gaining weight.
	› Client perception is that she is severely overweight and sees this image reflected in the mirror.
	› Client can exhibit low self-esteem, impulsivity, and difficulty with interpersonal relationships.
	› Client can exhibit the need for an intense physical regimen.
	› Client can experience guilt or shame due to binge-eating behavior.
Vital signs	› Low blood pressure with possible orthostatic hypotension.
	› Decreased pulse and body temperature.
	› Hypertension can be present in clients who have binge-eating disorder.
Weight	› Clients who have anorexia nervosa have a body weight less than 85% of expected normal weight.
	› Most clients who have bulimia nervosa maintain a weight within the normal range or slightly higher.
	› Clients who have binge-eating disorder are typically overweight or obese.
Skin, hair, and nails	› Clients who have anorexia nervosa can have fine, downy hair (lanugo) on the face and back; yellowed skin; mottled, cool extremities; and poor skin turgor.
Head, neck, mouth, and throat	› Enlargement of the parotid glands
	› Dental erosion and caries (if the client is purging)
Cardiovascular system	› Irregular heart rate (dysrhythmias noted on cardiac monitor), heart failure, cardiomyopathy
	› Peripheral edema
Musculoskeletal system	› Muscle weakness
Gastrointestinal system	› Constipation
	› Self-induced vomiting
	› Excessive use of diuretics or laxatives

- ○ Criteria for acute care treatment
  - Rapid weight loss or weight loss greater than 30% of body weight over 6 months
  - Unsuccessful weight gain in outpatient treatment, failure to adhere to treatment contract
  - Vital signs demonstrating heart rate less than 40/min, systolic blood pressure less than 70 mm Hg, body temperature less than 36° C (96.8° F)
  - ECG changes
  - Electrolyte disturbances
  - Psychiatric criteria – severe depression, suicidal behavior, family crisis, psychosis
- ○ Laboratory and diagnostic tests

  - Common laboratory abnormalities associated with anorexia
    - □ Hypokalemia, especially for those who have bulimia nervosa
      - ‣ There is a direct loss of potassium due to purging (vomiting).
      - ‣ Dehydration stimulates increased aldosterone production, which leads to sodium and water retention and potassium excretion.
    - □ Anemia and leukopenia with lymphocytosis
    - □ Possible impaired liver function, evidenced by increased enzyme levels
    - □ Possible elevated cholesterol
    - □ Abnormal thyroid function tests
    - □ Elevated carotene levels, which cause skin to appear yellow
    - □ Decreased bone density (possible osteoporosis)
    - □ Abnormal blood glucose level
    - □ ECG changes
  - Electrolyte imbalances associated with bulimia nervosa are common and can depend on the client's method of purging (laxatives, diuretics, vomiting). Laboratory abnormalities include the following.
    - □ Hypokalemia
    - □ Hyponatremia
    - □ Hypochloremia
- ○ Standardized screening tools
  - Eating Disorders Inventory
  - Body Attitude Test
  - Diagnostic Survey for Eating Disorders
  - Eating Attitudes Test

Patient-Centered Care

- Nursing Care
  - Perform self-assessment regarding possible feelings of frustration regarding client eating behaviors, the belief that the disorder is self-imposed, or the need to nurture rather than care for the client.
  - Provide a highly structured milieu in an acute care unit for the client requiring intensive therapy.
  - Develop and maintain a trusting nurse/client relationship through consistency and therapeutic communication.
  - Use a positive approach and support to promote client self-esteem and positive self-image.
  - Encourage client decision-making and participation in the plan of care to allow for a sense of control.
  - Establish realistic goals for weight loss or gain.

  - Promote cognitive-behavioral therapies.
    - Cognitive reframing
    - Relaxation techniques
    - Journal writing
    - Desensitization exercises
  - Monitor vital signs, intake and output, and weight.
  - Use behavioral contracts to modify client behaviors.
  - Reward the client for positive behaviors, such as completing meals or consuming a set number of calories.
  - Closely monitor the client during and after meals to prevent purging, which can necessitate accompanying the client to the bathroom.
  - Monitor the client for maintenance of appropriate exercise.
  - Discuss and encourage self-care activities.
  - Incorporate the family when appropriate in client education and discharge planning.
  - Work with a dietitian to provide nutrition education to include correcting misinformation regarding food, meal planning, and food selection.
    - Consider the client's preferences and ability to consume food when developing the initial eating plan.
    - A structured and inflexible eating schedule at the start of therapy, only permitting food during scheduled times, promotes new eating habits and discourages binge or binge-purge behavior.
    - Provide small, frequent meals, which are better tolerated and will help prevent the client from feeling overwhelmed.
    - Provide a diet high in fiber to prevent constipation.
    - Provide a diet low in sodium to prevent fluid retention.
    - Limit high-fat and gassy foods during the start of treatment.
    - Administer a multivitamin and mineral supplement.
    - Tell the client to avoid caffeine to reduce the risk for increased energy, resulting in difficulty controlling eating disorder behaviors. Caffeine also can be used by clients as a substitute for healthy eating.
  - Make arrangements for the client to attend individual, group, and family therapy to assist in resolving personal issues contributing to the eating disorder.

- Medications
  - Selective serotonin reuptake inhibitors (SSRIs), such as fluoxetine (Prozac)
    - Nursing Considerations
      - □ Tell the client that medication can take 1 to 3 weeks for initial response, with up to 2 months for maximal response.
      - □ Encourage the client to avoid hazardous activities (driving, operating heavy equipment/machinery) until individual side effects are known.
      - □ Tell the client to notify the provider if sexual dysfunction occurs and is intolerable.
- Teamwork and Collaboration
  - A registered dietitian should be involved to provide the client with nutritional and dietary guidance.
  - Consistency of care among all staff is important.
- Care After Discharge
  - Assist the client to develop and implement a maintenance plan related to weight management.
  - Encourage follow-up treatment in an outpatient setting.
  - Encourage client participation in a support group.
  - Continue individual and family therapy as indicated.
- Complications
  - Refeeding syndrome – the potentially fatal complication that can occur when fluids, electrolytes, and carbohydrates are introduced to a severely malnourished client
    - Nursing actions
      - □ Care for the client in a hospital setting.
      - □ Consult with the provider and dietitian to develop a controlled rate of nutritional support during initial treatment.
      - □ Monitor serum electrolytes, and administer fluid replacement.

  - Cardiac dysrhythmias, severe bradycardia, and hypotension
    - Nursing actions
      - □ Place the client on continuous cardiac monitoring.
      - □ Monitor vital signs frequently.
      - □ Report changes in the client's status to the provider.

APPLICATION EXERCISES

1. A nurse is preparing to obtain a nursing history from a client who has a new diagnosis of anorexia nervosa. Which of the following questions are appropriate for the nurse to include in the data collection? (Select all that apply.)

_____ A. "What is your relationship like with your family?"

_____ B. "Why do you want to lose weight?"

_____ C. "Would you describe your current eating habits?"

_____ D. "At what weight do you believe you will look better?"

_____ E. "Can you discuss your feelings about your appearance?"

2. A nurse is caring for an adolescent client who has anorexia nervosa with recent rapid weight loss and a current weight of 90 lb. Which of the following statements indicates the client is experiencing the cognitive distortion of catastrophizing?

A. "Life isn't worth living if I gain weight."

B. "Don't pretend like you don't know how fat I am."

C. "If I could be skinny, I know I'd be popular."

D. "When I look in the mirror, I see myself as obese."

3. A nurse is assisting a charge nurse with an admission assessment of a client who has bulimia nervosa with purging behavior. Which of the following are expected findings? (Select all that apply.)

_____ A. Hyponatremia

_____ B. Hypokalemia

_____ C. Mottling of the skin

_____ D. Slightly elevated body weight

_____ E. Presence of lanugo on the face

4. A nurse is caring for a client who has bulimia nervosa and who has stopped purging behavior. The client tells the nurse that she is afraid she is going to gain weight. Which of the following is an appropriate response by the nurse?

    A. "Many clients are concerned about their weight. However, the dietitian will ensure that you don't get too many calories in your diet."

    B. "Instead of worrying about your weight, try to focus on other problems at this time."

    C. "I understand you have concerns about your weight, but first, let's talk about your recent accomplishments."

    D. "You are not overweight, and the staff will ensure that you do not gain weight while you are in the hospital. We know that is important to you."

5. A nurse on an acute care unit is assisting with planning care for a client who has anorexia nervosa with binge-eating and purging behavior. Which of the following nursing actions is appropriate to include in the client's plan of care?

    A. Allow the client to select preferred meal times.

    B. Establish consequences for purging behavior.

    C. Provide the client with a high-fat diet at the start of treatment.

    D. Implement one-to-one observation during meal times.

6. A nurse is caring for a client who has anorexia nervosa of the restricting type. The client refuses to eat and exhibits severe anxiety when food is offered. The nurse plans to use desensitization as a behavioral therapy. Use the ATI Active Learning Template: Therapeutic Procedure to complete this item. Include the following:

    A. Description of Procedure

    B. Indications

    C. Nursing Actions: Identify at least two.

APPLICATION EXERCISES KEY

1. A. **CORRECT:** A nursing history of a client who has anorexia nervosa should include information regarding of family and interpersonal relationships.

   B. INCORRECT: Asking a "why" question promotes a defensive client response and is nontherapeutic.

   C. **CORRECT:** A nursing history of a client who has anorexia nervosa should include the client's current eating habits.

   D. INCORRECT: This question promotes cognitive distortion, places the focus on weight, and implies that the client's current appearance is not acceptable.

   E. **CORRECT:** A nursing history of a client who has anorexia nervosa should include the client's perception of the issue.

   Ⓝ NCLEX® Connection: Psychosocial Integrity, Mental Health Concepts

2. A. **CORRECT:** This statement reflects the cognitive distortion of catastrophizing because the client's perception of her appearance or situation is much worse than her current condition.

   B. INCORRECT: This statement reflects the cognitive distortion of personalization.

   C. INCORRECT: This statement reflects the cognitive distortion of overgeneralization.

   D. INCORRECT: This statement reflects a perception of distorted body image commonly experienced by the client who has anorexia nervosa. However, it is not an example of catastrophizing.

   Ⓝ NCLEX® Connection: Psychosocial Integrity, Mental Health Concepts

3. A. **CORRECT:** Hyponatremia is an expected finding of purging-type bulimia nervosa.

   B. **CORRECT:** Hypokalemia is an expected finding of purging-type bulimia nervosa.

   C. INCORRECT: Mottling of the skin is an expected finding of anorexia nervosa rather than bulimia nervosa.

   D. **CORRECT:** Most clients who have bulimia nervosa maintain a weight within a normal range or slightly higher.

   E. INCORRECT: Lanugo is an expected finding of anorexia nervosa rather than bulimia nervosa.

   Ⓝ NCLEX® Connection: Basic Care and Comfort, Nutrition and Oral Hydration

4. A. INCORRECT: This statement minimizes and generalizes the client's concern and is therefore a nontherapeutic response.

    B. INCORRECT: This statement minimizes the client's concern and is therefore a nontherapeutic response.

    C. **CORRECT:** This statement acknowledges the client's concern and then focuses the conversation on the client's accomplishments, which can promote client self-esteem and self-image.

    D. INCORRECT: This statement minimizes the client's concern and is therefore a nontherapeutic response.

    Ⓝ NCLEX® Connection: Psychosocial Integrity, Mental Health Concepts

5. A. INCORRECT: The nurse should provide a highly structured milieu, including meal times, for the client requiring acute care for the treatment of anorexia nervosa.

    B. INCORRECT: The nurse should use a positive approach to client care that includes rewards rather than consequences.

    C. INCORRECT: The nurse should limit high-fat and gas-producing foods at the start of treatment.

    D. **CORRECT:** The nurse should closely monitor the client during and after meals to prevent purging.

    Ⓝ NCLEX® Connection: Psychosocial Integrity, Mental Health Concepts

6. *Using the ATI Active Learning Template: Therapeutic Procedure*

    A. Description of Procedure
        *   Systematic desensitization is the planned, progressive, or graduated exposure to anxiety-provoking stimuli. During exposure, the anxiety response is suppressed through the use of relaxation techniques.

    B. Indications
        *   Systematic desensitization is appropriate for clients who have anorexia nervosa and anxiety related to food and eating.

    C. Nursing Actions
        *   Provide the client with relaxation techniques.
        *   Gradually expose the client to food starting with small amounts of a food.
        *   Stay with the client during meals to assist with relaxation.
        *   Reward the client for food intake.
        *   Use a positive approach to communicate the procedure and expectations to the client.

    Ⓝ NCLEX® Connection: Psychosocial Integrity, Behavioral Management

UNIT 4 Psychopharmacological Therapies

CHAPTERS

› Medications for Anxiety Disorders
› Medications for Depressive Disorders
› Medications for Bipolar Disorders
› Medications for Psychotic Disorders
› Medications for Children and Adolescents with Mental Health Issues
› Medications for Substance Use Disorders

NCLEX® CONNECTIONS

When reviewing the chapters in this unit, keep in mind the relevant sections of the NCLEX® outline, in particular:

Client Needs: Pharmacological Therapies

› Relevant topics/tasks include:
  » Adverse Effects/Contraindications/Side Effects/Interactions
   › Monitor for anticipated interactions among the client's prescribed medications and fluids.
  » Expected Actions/Outcomes
   › Evaluate the client's response to medications (adverse reactions, interactions, therapeutic effects).
  » Medication Administration
   › Collect required data prior to medication administration.

chapter 19

Overview

- The major medications used to treat anxiety disorders
  - Benzodiazepine sedative hypnotic anxiolytics, such as alprazolam (Xanax)
  - Atypical anxiolytic/nonbarbiturate anxiolytics, such as buspirone
  - Selected antidepressants such as
    - Paroxetine (Paxil), a selective serotonin reuptake inhibitor (SSRI)
    - Sertraline (Zoloft), an SSRI
    - Venlafaxine, a serotonin-norepinephrine reuptake inhibitor (SNRI)
- Other classifications that may be used
  - Other antidepressants
    - Amitriptyline, a tricyclic antidepressant (TCA)
    - Clomipramine (Anafranil), a TCA
  - Antihistamines, such as hydroxyzine pamoate (Vistaril) and hydroxyzine hydrochloride (Atarax)
  - Beta blockers, such as propranolol (Inderal)
  - Anticonvulsants, such as gabapentin (Neurontin)
- In addition to anxiety disorders, these medications are used to treat trauma- and stressor-related disorders as well as obsessive-compulsive and related disorders.

MEDICATION CLASSIFICATION: BENZODIAZEPINE SEDATIVE HYPNOTIC ANXIOLYTICS

- Select Prototype Medication: alprazolam (Xanax)
- Other Medications
  - Diazepam (Valium)
  - Lorazepam (Ativan)
  - Chlordiazepoxide (Librium)
  - Clorazepate (Tranxene)
  - Oxazepam (Serax)
  - Clonazepam (Klonopin)

Purpose

- Expected Pharmacological Action
  - Diazepam enhances the inhibitory effects of gamma-aminobutyric acid (GABA) in the central nervous system. Relief from anxiety occurs rapidly following administration.
- Therapeutic Uses
  - Generalized anxiety disorder and panic disorder
  - Other uses for benzodiazepines
    - Seizure disorders
    - Insomnia
    - Muscle spasm
    - Alcohol withdrawal (for prevention and treatment of acute effects)
    - Induction of anesthesia
    - Amnesic prior to surgery or procedures

Complications

ADVERSE EFFECTS	NURSING INTERVENTIONS/CLIENT EDUCATION
› CNS depression, such as sedation, lightheadedness, ataxia, and decreased cognitive function	› Advise the client to observe for manifestations. Instruct the client to notify the provider if effects occur. › Advise the client to avoid hazardous activities (driving, operating heavy equipment/machinery).
› Anterograde amnesia – difficulty recalling events that occur after dosing	› Advise the client to observe for manifestations. Instruct the client to notify the provider and withhold the medication if effects occur.
› Acute toxicity » Oral toxicity – drowsiness, lethargy, confusion	› Advise the client and family to watch for manifestations of overdose. Notify the provider if these occur. › For oral toxicity, gastric lavage is used, followed by the administration of activated charcoal or saline cathartics. › Flumazenil is administered to counteract sedation and reverse the adverse effects. › Monitor the client's vital signs, maintain patent airway, and provide fluids to maintain blood pressure. › Ensure availability of resuscitation equipment.
› Paradoxical response (insomnia, excitation, euphoria, anxiety, rage)	› Advise the client to observe for indications. Instruct the client to notify the provider if paradoxical response occurs.
› Withdrawal effects include anxiety, insomnia, diaphoresis, tremors, and lightheadedness. Withdrawal occurs infrequently with short-term use.	› After taking diazepam regularly and in high doses, the client should taper the dose over several weeks using a prescribed tapered dosing schedule.

Contraindications/Precautions

- Alprazolam is a Pregnancy Risk Category D medication.
- Benzodiazepines are classified under Schedule IV of the Controlled Substances Act.
- Alprazolam is contraindicated in clients who have pulmonary disease, myasthenia gravis, or glaucoma.
- Use alprazolam cautiously in clients who have liver disease or a history of alcohol use disorder.
- Benzodiazepines are generally used short-term due to the risk for dependence.

Medication/Food Interactions

MEDICATION/FOOD INTERACTIONS	NURSING INTERVENTIONS/CLIENT EDUCATION
› CNS depressants, such as alcohol, barbiturates, and opioids can cause respiratory depression.	› Advise the client to avoid alcohol and other substances that cause CNS depression. › Advise the client to avoid hazardous activities (driving, operating heavy equipment/machinery).

Nursing Administration

- Advise the client to take the medication as prescribed, and to avoid abrupt discontinuation of treatment to prevent withdrawal manifestations.
- When discontinuing benzodiazepines that have been taken regularly for long periods and in higher doses, taper the dose over several weeks using a prescribed dosing schedule.
- Administer the medication with meals or snacks if GI upset occurs.
- Advise the client to swallow sustained-release tablets and to avoid chewing or crushing the tablets.
- Instruct the client about the potential for dependency during and after treatment and to notify the provider if indications of withdrawal occur.

MEDICATION CLASSIFICATION: ATYPICAL ANXIOLYTIC/NONBARBITURATE ANXIOLYTICS

- Select Prototype Medication: buspirone

Purpose

- Expected Pharmacological Action
  - The exact antianxiety mechanism of this medication is unknown. This medication does bind to serotonin and dopamine receptors. There is less potential for dependency than with other anxiolytics, and use of buspirone does not result in sedation or potentiate the effects of other CNS depressants.

- Therapeutic Uses
  - Panic disorder
  - Obsessive-compulsive and related disorders
  - Social anxiety disorder
  - Trauma- and stressor-related disorders, such as posttraumatic stress disorder (PTSD)

Complications

ADVERSE EFFECTS	NURSING INTERVENTIONS/CLIENT EDUCATION
› CNS effects, such as dizziness, nausea, headache, lightheadedness, agitation	› Advise clients to take with food to decrease nausea. › Because this medication does not cause sedation there is less risk for interference with physical activities.

Contraindications/Precautions

- Buspirone is a Pregnancy Risk Category B medication.
- Buspirone is not recommended for use by women who are breastfeeding.
- Use buspirone cautiously in older adult clients, as well as clients who have liver or kidney dysfunction.
- Buspirone is contraindicated for concurrent use with MAOI antidepressants, or for 14 days after MAOIs are discontinued. Hypertensive crisis can result.

Medication/Food Interactions

MEDICATION/FOOD INTERACTIONS	NURSING INTERVENTIONS/CLIENT EDUCATION
› Erythromycin, ketoconazole, St. John's wort, and grapefruit juice can increase the effects of buspirone.	› Advise the client to avoid the use of erythromycin and ketoconazole. › Advise clients to avoid herbal preparations containing St. John's wort. › Advise the client to avoid drinking grapefruit juice.

Nursing Administration

- Advise the client to take the medication with meals to prevent gastric irritation.
- Advise the client that effects do not occur immediately. It can take a week to notice first therapeutic effects, and 3 to 6 weeks to reach full therapeutic benefit. Medication should be taken on a regular basis, rather than an as-needed basis.
- Instruct clients that tolerance, dependence, or withdrawal manifestations are not an issue with this medication.

MEDICATION CLASSIFICATION:
SELECTIVE SEROTONIN REUPTAKE INHIBITORS (SSRIs)

- Select Prototype Medication: paroxetine (Paxil)
- Other Medications
  - Sertraline (Zoloft)
  - Escitalopram (Lexapro)
  - Fluoxetine (Prozac)
  - Fluvoxamine

Purpose

- Expected Pharmacological Action
  - Paroxetine selectively inhibits serotonin reuptake, allowing more serotonin to stay at the junction of the neurons.
  - It does not block uptake of dopamine or norepinephrine.
  - Paroxetine causes CNS stimulation, which can cause insomnia.
  - The medication has a long effective half-life. Up to 4 weeks are necessary to produce therapeutic medication levels.
- Therapeutic Uses
  - SSRI antidepressants are the first-line treatment for trauma- and stressor-related disorders.
  - Paroxetine
    - Generalized anxiety disorder (GAD)
    - Panic disorder – decreases both the frequency and intensity of panic attacks; also prevents anticipatory anxiety about attacks
    - Obsessive compulsive disorder (OCD) – reduces manifestations by increasing serotonin
    - Social anxiety disorder
    - Trauma- and stressor-related disorders
    - Depressive disorders
  - Sertraline is indicated for panic disorder, OCD, social anxiety disorder, and PTSD.
  - Escitalopram is indicated for GAD and OCD.
  - Fluoxetine is used for panic disorder and GAD.
  - Fluvoxamine is used for OCD and social anxiety disorder.

Complications

ADVERSE EFFECTS	NURSING INTERVENTIONS/CLIENT EDUCATION
› Early adverse effects (first few days/weeks): nausea, diaphoresis, tremor, fatigue, drowsiness	› Instruct the client to report adverse effects to the provider. › Instruct the client to take the medication as prescribed. › Advise the client that these effects should soon subside.
› Later adverse effects (after 5 to 6 weeks of therapy): sexual dysfunction (impotence, delayed or absent orgasm, delayed or absent ejaculation, decreased sexual interest), weight gain, headache	› Instruct the client to report problems with sexual function (managed with dose reduction, medication holiday, changing medications).
› Weight gain: 20 lb or more possible with long-term use of SSRIs	› Advise the client to follow a well-balanced diet and exercise regularly.
› Gastrointestinal bleeding	› Use cautiously in clients who have a history of gastrointestinal bleed, ulcers, and those taking other medications that affect blood coagulation. › Advise the client to report indications of bleeding, such as dark stools or emesis that has the appearance of coffee grounds.
› Hyponatremia – more likely in older adult clients taking diuretics	› Obtain baseline serum sodium, and monitor level periodically throughout treatment.
› Serotonin syndrome » Agitation, confusion, disorientation, difficulty concentrating, anxiety, hallucinations, hyperreflexia, fever, diaphoresis, incoordination, tremors » Usually begins 2 to 72 hr after initiation of treatment » Resolves when the medication is discontinued	› Watch for and advise the client to report any of these manifestations, which could indicate a lethal problem.
› Bruxism: grinding and clenching of teeth, usually during sleep	› Report bruxism to the provider, who may: » Switch the client to another class of medication. » Treat bruxism with low-dose buspirone. » Advise the client to use a mouth guard during sleep.
› Withdrawal syndrome » Nausea, sensory disturbances, anxiety, tremor, malaise, unease » Minimized by tapering the medication slowly	› Advise the client that, after a long period of use, taper the medication slowly according to a prescribed tapered dosing schedule to avoid withdrawal effects. › Advise the client to avoid abrupt discontinuation of the medication.

Contraindications/Precautions

- Paroxetine is a Pregnancy Risk Category D medication. Other SSRIs pose less risk during pregnancy.
- Paroxetine is contraindicated in clients taking MAOIs.
- Clients taking paroxetine should avoid alcohol.
- Use paroxetine cautiously in clients who have liver and kidney dysfunction, seizure disorders, or a history of gastrointestinal bleeding.

- Use SSRIs cautiously in clients who have bipolar disorder, due to the risk for mania.

Medication/Food Interactions

MEDICATION/FOOD INTERACTIONS	NURSING INTERVENTIONS/CLIENT EDUCATION
› Concurrent use of MAOIs or tricyclic antidepressants with paroxetine can cause serotonin syndrome.	› Advise the client to avoid concurrent use of these medications.

Nursing Administration

- Advise the client that paroxetine may be taken with food. Sleep disturbances are minimized by taking the medication in the morning.
- Instruct the client to take the medication on a daily basis to establish therapeutic plasma levels.
- Assist the client with medication regimen adherence by informing the client that it may take up to 4 weeks to achieve therapeutic effects.

Nursing Evaluation of Medication Effectiveness

- Depending on therapeutic intent, effectiveness is evidenced by:
  - Maintenance of a normal sleep pattern.
  - Verbalization of feeling less anxious and more relaxed.
  - Greater ability to participate in social and occupational interactions.

APPLICATION EXERCISES

1. A nurse working in a mental health clinic is reinforcing teaching with a client who has a new prescription for diazepam (Valium) for generalized anxiety disorder. Which of the following is appropriate for the nurse to include in the teaching?

    A. 3 to 6 weeks of treatment is required to achieve therapeutic benefit.

    B. Combining alcohol with diazepam will produce a paradoxical response.

    C. Diazepam has a lower risk for dependency than other antianxiety medications.

    D. Report confusion as a potential indication of toxicity.

2. A nurse is caring for a client who has benzodiazepine toxicity due to an overdose. Which of the following is the priority nursing action?

    A. Assist with the administration of flumazenil.

    B. Identify the client's level of orientation.

    C. Administer a saline cathartic.

    D. Prepare the client for gastric lavage.

3. A nurse is caring for a client who is to begin taking fluoxetine (Prozac) for treatment of generalized anxiety disorder. Which of the following statements indicates the client understands the use of this medication?

    A. "I will take the medication at bedtime."

    B. "I will follow a low-sodium diet while taking this medication."

    C. "I will need to discontinue this medication slowly."

    D. "I will be at risk for weight loss with long-term use of this medication."

4. A nurse is collecting data from a client 4 hr after receiving an initial dose of fluoxetine (Prozac). Which of the following findings should the nurse report to the provider as an indication of serotonin syndrome? (Select all that apply.)

    _____ A. Hypothermia

    _____ B. Hallucinations

    _____ C. Muscular flaccidity

    _____ D. Diaphoresis

    _____ E. Agitation

5. A nurse is caring for a client who takes paroxetine (Paxil) to treat posttraumatic stress disorder. The client states that he grinds his teeth during the night which causes pain in his mouth. The nurse should identify which of the following as possible measures to manage the client's bruxism? (Select all that apply.)

_____ A. Concurrent administration of buspirone

_____ B. Administration of a different SSRI

_____ C. Use of a mouth guard

_____ D. Changing to a different class of antianxiety medication

_____ E. Increasing the dose of paroxetine

6. A nurse is reinforcing teaching with a client who has a new prescription for buspirone. Use the ATI Active Learning Template: Medication to complete this item to include the following sections:

A. Therapeutic Uses: Identify at least three therapeutic uses for this medication.

B. Side/Adverse Effects: List at least three adverse effects of this medication.

C. Medication/Food Interactions: Identify two medication and one food interaction.

D. Nursing Interventions/Client Education: Describe two things to reinforce with the client to reduce the risk of medication/food interactions.

APPLICATION EXERCISES KEY

1. A. INCORRECT: Buspirone, rather than diazepam, requires 3 to 6 weeks to achieve therapeutic benefit.

    B. INCORRECT: Combining alcohol with diazepam can produce CNS and respiratory depression, rather than a paradoxical response.

    C. INCORRECT: Diazepam is preferably used for short-term treatment because of the increased risk of dependency.

    D. **CORRECT:** Confusion is a potential indication of diazepam toxicity that the client should report to the provider.

    (N) NCLEX® Connection: Pharmacological Therapies, Adverse Effects/Contraindications/ Side Effects/Interactions

2. A. INCORRECT: Assisting with the administration of flumazenil is an appropriate action. However, it is not the priority when taking the nursing process approach to client care.

    B. **CORRECT:** When taking the nursing process approach to client care, the initial step is data collection. Therefore, identifying the client's level of orientation is the priority action.

    C. INCORRECT: Administration of a saline cathartic is an appropriate action. However, it is not the priority when taking the nursing process approach to client care.

    D. INCORRECT: Gastric lavage is an appropriate action. However, it is not the priority when taking the nursing process approach to client care.

    (N) NCLEX® Connection: Psychosocial Integrity, Chemical and Other Dependencies

3. A. INCORRECT: The client should take fluoxetine in the morning to minimize sleep disturbances.

    B. INCORRECT: The client is at risk for hyponatremia while taking fluoxetine.

    C. **CORRECT:** When discontinuing fluoxetine, the client should taper the medication slowly according to a prescribed tapered dosing schedule to reduce the risk of withdrawal syndrome.

    D. INCORRECT: The client is at risk for weight gain, rather than loss, with long-term use of fluoxetine.

    (N) NCLEX® Connection: Pharmacological Therapies, Medication Administration

4. A. INCORRECT: Fever, rather than hypothermia, is an indication of serotonin syndrome.

    B. **CORRECT:** Hallucinations are an indication of serotonin syndrome.

    C. INCORRECT: Muscle tremors, rather than flaccidity, are an indication of serotonin syndrome.

    D. **CORRECT:** Diaphoresis is an indication of serotonin syndrome.

    E. **CORRECT:** Agitation is an indication of serotonin syndrome.

    (N) NCLEX® Connection: Pharmacological Therapies, Adverse Effects/Contraindications/ Side Effects/Interactions

5. A. **CORRECT:** Concurrent administration of a low-dose of buspirone is an effective measure to manage the adverse effect of paroxetine.

    B. INCORRECT: Other SSRIs also have bruxism as an adverse effect. Therefore, this is not an effective measure.

    C. **CORRECT:** Using a mouth guard during sleep can decrease the risk for oral damage resulting from bruxism.

    D. **CORRECT:** Changing to different class of antianxiety medication that does not have the adverse effect of bruxism is an effective measure.

    E. INCORRECT: Increasing the dose of paroxetine can cause the adverse effect of bruxism to worsen. Therefore, this is not an effective measure.

    (N) NCLEX® Connection: Physiological Adaptations, Alterations in Body Systems

6. *Using the ATI Active Learning Template: Medication*

    A. Therapeutic Uses
    - Panic disorder
    - Obsessive-compulsive and related disorders
    - Social anxiety disorder
    - Trauma- and stressor-related disorders

    B. Side/Adverse Effects
    - Dizziness
    - Nausea
    - Headache
    - Lightheadedness
    - Agitation

    C. Medication/Food Interactions
    - Medication Interaction
      - MAOI antidepressants
      - Erythromycin
      - Ketoconazole
    - Food Interaction
      - Grapefruit juice

    D. Nursing Interventions/Client Education
    - Buspirone is contraindicated for concurrent use with MAOI antidepressants, or for 14 days after MAOIs are discontinued due to the risk for hypertensive crisis.
    - Avoid the use of erythromycin or ketoconazole, which can increase the effects of buspirone.
    - Avoid drinking grapefruit juice, which can increase the effects of buspirone.

    (N) NCLEX® Connection: Pharmacological Therapies, Expected Actions/Outcomes

chapter 20

Overview

- Depressive disorders affect many clients and are a leading cause of disability.
- Advise clients starting antidepressant medication therapy for a depressive disorder that relief is not immediate, and it can take several weeks or more to reach full therapeutic benefits. Encourage continued compliance.
- Clients who have major depression can require hospitalization with the implementation of close observation and suicide precautions until antidepressant medications reach their peak effect.
- Antidepressant medications are classified into four main groups.
  - Tricyclic antidepressants (TCAs)
  - Selective serotonin reuptake inhibitors (SSRIs)
  - Monoamine oxidase inhibitors (MAOIs)
  - Atypical antidepressants

MEDICATION CLASSIFICATION: TRICYCLIC ANTIDEPRESSANTS (TCAs)

- Select Prototype Medication: amitriptyline
- Other Medications
  - Imipramine (Tofranil)
  - Doxepin (Prudoxin)
  - Nortriptyline (Aventyl, Pamelor)
  - Amoxapine
  - Trimipramine (Surmontil)

Purpose

- Expected Pharmacological Action
  - These medications block reuptake of norepinephrine and serotonin in the synaptic space, thereby intensifying the effects of these neurotransmitters.
- Therapeutic Uses
  - Depressive disorders
- Other Uses
  - Neuropathic pain
  - Fibromyalgia
  - Anxiety disorders
  - Insomnia

Complications

ADVERSE EFFECTS	NURSING INTERVENTIONS/CLIENT EDUCATION
› Orthostatic hypotension	› Instruct the client about the indications of postural hypotension (lightheadedness, dizziness). If these occur, advise the client to sit or lie down. Orthostatic hypotension is minimized by getting up or changing positions slowly. › Monitor the hospitalized client's blood pressure and heart rate for orthostatic changes. If a significant decrease in blood pressure and/or increase in heart rate is noted, do not administer the medication and notify the provider. › Advise the client to avoid dehydration, which increases the risk for hypotension.
› Anticholinergic effects » Dry mouth » Blurred vision » Photophobia » Urinary hesitancy or retention » Constipation » Tachycardia	› Instruct the client on ways to minimize anticholinergic effects. » Chewing sugarless gum » Sipping on water » Wearing sunglasses when outdoors » Eating foods high in fiber » Exercising regularly to promote peristalsis » Increasing fluid intake to at least 2 L/day from beverage and food sources » Voiding just before taking the medication › Advise the client to notify the provider if adverse effects persist.
› Sedation	› This adverse effect usually diminishes over time. › Advise the client to avoid hazardous activities, such as driving, if sedation is excessive. › Advise the client to take medication at bedtime to minimize daytime sleepiness and to promote sleep.
› Toxicity resulting in cholinergic blockade and cardiac toxicity evidenced by dysrhythmias, mental confusion, and agitation, which are followed by seizures, coma, and possible death	› Give no more than a 1-week supply of medication to clients who are acutely ill due to the high risk of lethality with overdose. › Obtain the client's baseline ECG. › Monitor vital signs frequently. › Monitor for indications of toxicity. › Notify the primary care provider if indications of toxicity occur.
› Decreased seizure threshold	› Monitor clients who have seizure disorders.
› Excessive sweating	› Inform the client of this adverse effect. › Assist the client with frequent linen changes.

Contraindications/Precautions

- Amitriptyline is a Pregnancy Risk Category C medication.

- This medication is contraindicated for clients who have seizure disorders.

- Use this medication cautiously in clients who have coronary artery disease; diabetes; liver, kidney, and respiratory disorders; urinary retention and obstruction; angle closure glaucoma; benign prostatic hypertrophy; and hyperthyroidism.

Medication/Food Interactions

MEDICATION/FOOD INTERACTIONS	NURSING INTERVENTIONS/ CLIENT EDUCATION
› Concurrent use with MAOIs can cause severe hypertension.	› Avoid concurrent use of TCAs and MAOIs.
› Concurrent use with antihistamines and other anticholinergic agents can result in additive anticholinergic effects.	› Avoid concurrent use of TCAs and antihistamines.
› Concurrent use with direct-acting sympathomimetics can result in increased effects of these medications, because uptake is blocked by TCAs.	› Avoid concurrent use of TCAs and these medications.
› Concurrent use with indirect-acting sympathomimetics can result in decreased effect of these medications, due to the inhibition of their uptake and inability to get to the site of action in the nerve terminal.	› Avoid concurrent use of TCAs and these medications.
› Concurrent use with alcohol, benzodiazepines, opioids, and antihistamines can result in additive CNS depression.	› Advise the client to avoid other CNS depressants.

MEDICATION CLASSIFICATION:
SELECTIVE SEROTONIN REUPTAKE INHIBITORS (SSRIs)

- Select Prototype Medication: fluoxetine (Prozac)
- Other Medications
  - Citalopram (Celexa)
  - Escitalopram (Lexapro)
  - Paroxetine (Paxil)
  - Sertraline (Zoloft)
  - Vilazodone (Viibryd)

Purpose

- Expected Pharmacological Action
  - SSRIs selectively block reuptake of the monoamine neurotransmitter serotonin in the synaptic space, thereby intensifying the effects of serotonin.
- Therapeutic Uses
  - Major depressive disorder
  - Obsessive compulsive disorder
  - Bulimia nervosa
  - Premenstrual dysphoric disorders
  - Panic disorders
  - Posttraumatic stress disorder (PTSD)

Complications

ADVERSE EFFECTS	NURSING INTERVENTIONS/CLIENT EDUCATION
› Sexual dysfunction (anorgasmia, impotence, decreased libido)	› Warn the client of possible adverse effects, and to notify the provider if they become intolerable.
	› Instruct the client on ways to manage sexual dysfunction, which may include lowering the dosage, discontinuing the medication temporarily (medication holiday), and using adjunct medications to improve sexual function.
	› Inform the client that the provider can prescribe an atypical antidepressant with fewer sexual dysfunction adverse effects, such as bupropion (Wellbutrin).
› CNS stimulation (insomnia, agitation, anxiety)	› Advise the client to notify the provider for a possible dosage reduction.
	› Advise the client to take this medication in the morning.
	› Advise the client to avoid caffeinated beverages.
	› Reinforce teaching for the client about relaxation techniques to promote sleep.

ADVERSE EFFECTS	NURSING INTERVENTIONS/CLIENT EDUCATION
› Occurrence of weight loss early in therapy that can be followed by weight gain with long-term treatment	› Monitor the client's weight. › Encourage the client to participate in regular exercise and to follow a healthy, well-balanced diet.
› Serotonin syndrome can begin 2 to 72 hr after the start of treatment, and it can be lethal. Manifestations include: » Mental confusion, difficulty concentrating » Abdominal pain » Diarrhea » Agitation » Fever » Anxiety » Hallucinations » Hyperreflexia, incoordination » Diaphoresis » Tremors	› Advise the client to observe for manifestations. If any occur, instruct the client to withhold the medication and notify the provider.
› Withdrawal syndrome (headache, nausea, visual disturbances, anxiety, dizziness, and tremors)	› Instruct the client to taper the dose gradually when discontinuing the medication using a prescribed tapered dosing schedule.
› Hyponatremia, which is more likely to occur in older adult clients taking diuretics	› Obtain a baseline serum sodium, and monitor the level periodically throughout treatment.
› Rash	› Advise the client that a rash is treatable with an antihistamine or discontinuation of the medication.
› Sleepiness, faintness, lightheadedness	› Advise the client that these adverse effects are not common, but can occur. › The client should avoid driving if these effects occur.
› Gastrointestinal bleeding	› Use cautiously in clients who have a history of gastrointestinal bleeding and ulcers, and in those taking other medications that affect blood coagulation.
› Bruxism	› Advise the client to report this to the provider. › Advise the client to use a mouth guard, and that changing to a different classification of antidepressants, or adding a low dose of buspirone, may decrease this adverse effect.

Contraindications/Precautions

- Fluoxetine is a Pregnancy Risk Category C medication.

- Fluoxetine and paroxetine can increase the risk of birth defects. Other SSRIs are recommended. Late in pregnancy, use of SSRIs can increase the risk of withdrawal effects or pulmonary hypertension in the newborn.

- These medications are contraindicated in clients taking MAOIs or TCAs.

- Use cautiously in clients who have liver or kidney dysfunction, cardiac disease, seizure disorders, diabetes mellitus, ulcers, and a history of gastrointestinal bleeding.

Medication/Food Interactions

MEDICATION/FOOD INTERACTIONS	NURSING INTERVENTIONS/CLIENT EDUCATION
› Concurrent use with MAOIs, TCAs, or St. John's wort increases the risk of serotonin syndrome.	› Discontinue MAOIs 14 days prior to starting an SSRI. Fluoxetine should be discontinued 5 weeks before starting an MAOI. › Advise the client against concurrent use of TCAs and St. John's wort along with SSRIs.
› Concurrent use with warfarin (Coumadin) can displace warfarin from bound protein and result in increased warfarin levels.	› Monitor prothrombin time (PT) and INR levels. › Monitor for indications of bleeding and the need for dosage adjustment.
› Concurrent use with TCAs and lithium may result in increased levels of these medications.	› Advise the client to avoid concurrent use.
› Concurrent use with NSAIDs and anticoagulants can further suppress platelet aggregation, thereby increasing the risk of bleeding.	› Advise the client to monitor for indications of bleeding (bruising, hematuria) and to notify the provider if they occur.

MEDICATION CLASSIFICATION: MONOAMINE OXIDASE INHIBITORS (MAOIs)

- Select Prototype Medication: phenelzine (Nardil)
- Other Medications
  - Isocarboxazid (Marplan)
  - Tranylcypromine (Parnate)
  - Selegiline (Emsam) – transdermal patch

Purpose

- Expected Pharmacological Action
  - These medications block MAO in the brain, thereby increasing the amount of norepinephrine, dopamine, and serotonin available for transmission of impulses. An increased amount of those neurotransmitters at nerve endings intensifies responses and relieves depression.
- Therapeutic Uses
  - Depression
  - Bulimia nervosa

Complications

ADVERSE EFFECTS	NURSING INTERVENTIONS/CLIENT EDUCATION
› CNS stimulation (e.g., anxiety, agitation, hypomania, mania)	› Advise the client to observe for effects and to notify the provider if they occur.
› Orthostatic hypotension	› Monitor the client's blood pressure and heart rate for orthostatic changes. › Hold the medication, and notify the provider regarding significant changes. › Advise the client to change positions slowly.
› Hypertensive crisis resulting from intake of dietary tyramine – severe hypertension as a result of intensive vasoconstriction and stimulation of the heart. Manifestations may include: » Headache » Nausea » Increased heart rate » Increased blood pressure	› Assist with emergency care.
› Local rash associated with transdermal preparation	› Choose a clean, dry area for each application. › Apply a topical glucocorticoid on the affected areas if rash occurs.

Contraindications/Precautions

- Phenelzine is a Pregnancy Risk Category C medication.
- MAOIs are contraindicated in clients taking SSRIs, or clients who have pheochromocytoma, heart failure, cardiovascular and cerebral vascular disease, or severe impairment of kidney function.
- Use cautiously in clients who have diabetes or seizure disorders, or those taking TCAs.
- Transdermal selegiline is contraindicated for clients taking carbamazepine (Tegretol) or oxcarbazepine (Trileptal). Concurrent use of these medications may increase blood levels of the MAOI.

Medication/Food Interactions

MEDICATION/FOOD INTERACTIONS	NURSING INTERVENTIONS/CLIENT EDUCATION
› Concurrent use with indirect-acting sympathomimetic medications (ephedrine, amphetamine) can promote the release of norepinephrine and lead to hypertensive crisis.	› Instruct the client that over-the-counter decongestants and cold remedies frequently contain medications with sympathomimetic action and therefore should be avoided.
› Concurrent use with TCAs can lead to hypertensive crisis.	› Avoid concurrent use of MAOIs and TCAs.
› Concurrent use with SSRIs can lead to serotonin syndrome.	› Avoid concurrent use.
› Concurrent use with antihypertensives can cause additive hypotensive effects.	› Monitor the client's blood pressure. › Notify the provider if there is a significant drop in the client's blood pressure, as the dosage of antihypertensive may need to be reduced.
› Concurrent use with meperidine (Demerol) can lead to hyperpyrexia.	› Alternative analgesic should be used.
› Hypertensive crisis (severe hypertension as a result of intensive vasoconstriction and stimulation of the heart) can result from intake of dietary tyramine. Manifestations can include: » Headache » Nausea » Increase heart rate » Increased blood pressure	› Determine the client's ability to follow strict adherence to dietary restrictions. › Inform the client of indications and to notify the provider if they occur. › Provide the client with written instructions regarding foods and beverages to avoid. › Tyramine-rich foods include aged meats and cheeses, smoked or pickled meats, meat extracts, avocado, smoked fish, some dietary supplements, some beers, and red wine. › Advise the client to avoid taking any medications (prescription or over-the-counter) without approval from the provider.
› Concurrent use with vasopressors (caffeine, phenylethylamine) can result in hypertension.	› Advise the client to avoid foods that contain these agents (caffeinated beverages, chocolate, fava beans, ginseng).

MEDICATION CLASSIFICATION: ATYPICAL ANTIDEPRESSANTS

- Select Prototype Medication: bupropion (Wellbutrin)

Purpose

- Expected Pharmacological Action
  - This medication acts by inhibiting dopamine uptake.
- Therapeutic Uses
  - Treatment of depression
  - Alternative to SSRIs for clients unable to tolerate the sexual dysfunction adverse effects
  - Aid to quit smoking
  - Prevention of seasonal affective disorder

Complications

ADVERSE EFFECTS	NURSING INTERVENTIONS/CLIENT EDUCATION
› Headache, dry mouth, GI distress, constipation, increased heart rate, nausea, restlessness, insomnia	› Advise the client to observe for effects and to notify the provider if they become intolerable. › Treat headaches with a mild analgesic. › Advise the client to sip water to treat dry mouth, and to increase dietary fiber to prevent constipation.
› Suppression of appetite resulting in weight loss	› Monitor the client's food intake and weight.
› Seizures, especially at higher dose ranges	› Avoid administering to clients at risk for seizures, such as a client who has a head injury. › Monitor for seizures, and treat accordingly.

Contraindications/Precautions

- Bupropion is a Pregnancy Risk Category B medication.
- This medication is contraindicated in clients who have a seizure disorder.
- This medication is contraindicated in clients taking MAOIs.
- Bupropion is contraindicated in clients who have anorexia nervosa or bulimia nervosa.

Medication/Food Interactions

MEDICATION/FOOD INTERACTIONS	NURSING INTERVENTIONS/CLIENT EDUCATION
› Concurrent use with MAOIs, such as phenelzine (Nardil), can increase the risk for toxicity.	› MAOIs should be discontinued 2 weeks prior to beginning treatment with bupropion.

OTHER ATYPICAL ANTIDEPRESSANTS

AGENT	PHARMACOLOGICAL ACTION	NURSING IMPLICATIONS
Venlafaxine, duloxetine (Cymbalta), desvenlafaxine (Pristiq)	› These agents inhibit serotonin and norepinephrine reuptake, thereby increasing the amount of these neurotransmitters available in the brain for impulse transmission. There is also a minimal amount of dopamine blockade.	› Adverse effects include headache, nausea, agitation, anxiety, and sleep disturbances. › Monitor for hyponatremia, especially in older adult clients. › Monitor for weight loss. › Monitor for increases in diastolic blood pressure. › Discuss ways to manage interference with sexual functioning. › Advise the client to avoid abrupt cessation of the medication.
Mirtazapine (Remeron)	› This agent increases the release of serotonin and norepinephrine, thereby increasing the amount of these neurotransmitters available for impulse transmission.	› Therapeutic effects can occur sooner, and with less sexual dysfunction, than with SSRIs. › This medication is generally well tolerated. Adverse effects include sleepiness that can be exacerbated by other CNS depressants, weight gain, and elevated cholesterol.
Trazodone (Oleptro)	› This agent has moderate selective blockade of serotonin receptors, thereby increasing the amount of that neurotransmitter available for impulse transmission.	› This agent is usually used with another antidepressant agent. Sedation may be an issue; therefore, it may be indicated for a client who has insomnia caused by an SSRI. Advise the client to take at bedtime. › Priapism can be a serious adverse effect, and clients should be instructed to seek medical attention immediately if this occurs.

Nursing Administration

- Instruct the client to take antidepressant medication as prescribed on a daily basis to establish therapeutic plasma levels.

- Assist with the client's medication regimen compliance by informing the client that therapeutic effects might not be experienced for 1 to 3 weeks. Full therapeutic effects can take 2 to 3 months.

- Instruct the client to continue therapy after improvement in manifestations. Sudden discontinuation of the medication can result in relapse.

- Advise the client that therapy usually continues for 6 months after resolution of manifestations, and it can continue for a year or longer.

- Suicide prevention is facilitated by prescribing only 1 week's worth of medication for an acutely ill client, and following that, only prescribing 1 month's worth of medication at a time, especially with TCAs, which have a high risk for lethality with overdose.

  - Collect data about the client's risk for suicide. Antidepressant medications can increase the client's risk for suicide, particularly during initial treatment. Antidepressant-induced suicide is mainly associated with clients under the age of 25.

- For TCAs:
  - Monitor for cardiac dysrhythmias, which are an indication of toxicity.
  - Administer at bedtime due to sedation and risk for orthostatic hypotension.
- For SSRIs:
  - Advise clients to take these medications in the morning to minimize sleep disturbances.
  - Advise clients to take these medications with food to minimize gastrointestinal disturbances.
  - Obtain baseline sodium levels for older adult clients taking diuretics. Monitor these clients periodically.
- For MAOIs:
  - Provide clients with a list of foods containing tyramine to reduce the risk of hypertensive crisis.
  - Instruct the client to avoid taking any other prescription or nonprescription medications unless approved by the provider.
- For atypical antidepressants:
  - Advise clients who have seasonal affective disorder to begin taking bupropion in autumn each year, gradually taper dose, and discontinue by spring.
  - Avoid concurrent use with MAOIs.

Nursing Evaluation of Medication Effectiveness

- Effectiveness of antidepressant medication can be evidenced by:
  - Verbalizing improvement in mood.
  - Ability to perform ADLs.
  - Improved sleeping and eating habits.
  - Increased interaction with peers.

APPLICATION EXERCISES

1. A nurse is reinforcing teaching with a client who has a new prescription for amitriptyline. Which of the following client statements indicates understanding of the teaching?

    A. "While taking this medication, I'll need to stay out of the sun to avoid a skin rash."

    B. "I may feel drowsy for a few weeks after starting this medication."

    C. "I cannot eat my favorite pizza with pepperoni while taking this medication."

    D. "This medication will help me lose the weight that I have gained over the last year."

2. A nurse is caring for a client who is taking phenelzine (Nardil). For which of the following adverse effects should the nurse observe? (Select all that apply.)

    _____ A. Elevated blood glucose level

    _____ B. Orthostatic hypotension

    _____ C. Priapism

    _____ D. Headache

    _____ E. Bruxism

3. A nurse is reviewing the medical record of a client who has a new prescription for bupropion (Wellbutrin) for depression. Which of the following findings is the priority for the nurse to report to the provider?

    A. The client has a family history of seasonal affective disorder.

    B. The client currently smokes 1.5 packs of cigarettes per day.

    C. The client had a motor vehicle crash last year and sustained a head injury.

    D. The client has a BMI of 25 and has gained 10 lb over the last year.

4. A charge nurse is discussing mirtazapine (Remeron) with a newly licensed nurse. Which of the following statements by the newly licensed nurse indicates understanding?

    A. "This medication increases the release of serotonin and norepinephrine."

    B. "I will need to monitor the client for hyponatremia while taking this medication."

    C. "This medication is contraindicated for clients who have an eating disorder."

    D. "Sexual dysfunction is a common adverse effect of this medication."

5. A nurse is reinforcing teaching with a client who has a new prescription for imipramine (Tofranil) about how to minimize anticholinergic effects. Which of the following should the nurse include in the teaching? (Select all that apply.)

_____ A. Void just before taking the medication.

_____ B. Increase the dietary intake of potassium.

_____ C. Wear sunglasses when outside.

_____ D. Change positions slowly when getting up.

_____ E. Chew sugarless gum.

6. A nurse is reinforcing teaching with a client who has a new prescription for sertraline (Zoloft) for the treatment of depression. Use the ATI Active Learning Template: Medication to complete this item to include the following sections:

A. Side/Adverse Effects: Identify at least four adverse effects of sertraline.

B. Medication/Food Interactions: Identify at least two interactions.

C. Nursing Administration: Identify two nursing administration interventions.

APPLICATION EXERCISES KEY

1. A. INCORRECT: Skin rash is associated with SSRIs, rather than TCAs like amitriptyline.

   B. **CORRECT:** Sedation is an adverse effect of amitriptyline during the first few weeks of therapy.

   C. INCORRECT: Foods such as pepperoni should be avoided if the client is prescribed an MAOI, rather than a TCA like amitriptyline.

   D. INCORRECT: Weight gain, rather than weight loss, is expected with TCAs.

   N NCLEX® Connection: Pharmacological Therapies, Adverse Effects/Contraindications/ Side Effects/Interactions

2. A. INCORRECT: An elevated blood glucose level is not an adverse effect of phenelzine.

   B. **CORRECT:** The nurse should observe for orthostatic hypotension, which is an adverse effect of phenelzine.

   C. INCORRECT: Priapism is an adverse effect of trazodone, rather than phenelzine.

   D. **CORRECT:** The nurse should observe for a headache, which is an adverse effect of phenelzine.

   E. INCORRECT: Bruxism is an adverse effect of SSRIs, rather than phenelzine.

   N NCLEX® Connection: Pharmacological Therapies, Adverse Effects/Contraindications/ Side Effects/Interactions

3. A. INCORRECT: The nurse should report family history information. However, this does not address the greatest risk to the client and is therefore not the priority.

   B. INCORRECT: The nurse should report the client's current smoking status. However, this does not address the greatest risk to the client and is therefore not the priority.

   C. **CORRECT:** The greatest risk to the client is development of seizures. Bupropion can lower the seizure threshold and should be avoided by clients who have a history of a head injury. This information is the priority to report to the provider.

   D. INCORRECT: The nurse should report the client's BMI and change in weight. However, this does not address the greatest risk to the client and is therefore not the priority.

   N NCLEX® Connection: Pharmacological Therapies, Adverse Effects/Contraindications/ Side Effects/Interactions

4. A. **CORRECT:** Mirtazapine provides relief from depression by increasing the release of serotonin and norepinephrine.

    B. INCORRECT: Hyponatremia is an adverse effect of venlafaxine, rather than mirtazapine.

    C. INCORRECT: Bupropion, rather than mirtazapine, is contraindicated in clients who have an eating disorder.

    D. INCORRECT: Sexual dysfunction is an adverse effect of SSRIs rather than mirtazapine.

    Ⓝ NCLEX® Connection: Pharmacological Therapies, Expected Actions/Outcomes

5. A. **CORRECT:** Voiding just before taking the medication will help minimize the anticholinergic effects of urinary hesitancy or retention.

    B. INCORRECT: The anticholinergic effects of imipramine do not affect the client's potassium level.

    C. **CORRECT:** Wearing sunglasses when outside will help minimize the anticholinergic effect of photophobia.

    D. INCORRECT: The client should change positions slowly to avoid orthostatic hypotension. However, this is not an anticholinergic effect.

    E. **CORRECT:** Chewing sugarless gum will help minimize the anticholinergic effect of dry mouth.

    Ⓝ NCLEX® Connection: Pharmacological Therapies, Adverse Effects/Contraindications/ Side Effects/Interactions

6. *Using the ATI Active Learning Template: Medication*

    A. Side/Adverse Effects
    - Sexual dysfunction
    - CNS stimulation
    - Weight changes
    - Serotonin syndrome
    - Hyponatremia
    - Rash
    - Gastrointestinal bleeding
    - Bruxism

    B. Medication/Food Interactions
    - MAOIs
    - TCAs
    - St. John's wort
    - Warfarin (Coumadin)
    - NSAIDs

    C. Nursing Administration
    - Administer SSRIs in the morning to minimize sleep disturbances.
    - Administer SSRIs with food to minimize gastrointestinal disturbances.
    - Instruct the client to take this medication on a daily basis.
    - Inform the client that therapeutic effects can take several weeks.

    Ⓝ NCLEX® Connection: Pharmacological Therapies, Adverse Effects/Contraindications/ Side Effects/Interactions

chapter 21

Overview

- Bipolar disorder is primarily managed with mood-stabilizing medications, such as lithium carbonate (Lithobid).

- Bipolar disorder also can be treated with some antiepileptic medications.

   ○ Valproic acid (Depakote)

   ○ Carbamazepine (Tegretol)

   ○ Lamotrigine (Lamictal)

- Other medications used for bipolar disorder include the following.

   ○ Atypical antipsychotics – These can be useful in early treatment to promote sleep and to decrease anxiety and agitation. These medications also demonstrate mood-stabilizing properties.

   ○ Anxiolytics – Clonazepam (Klonopin) and lorazepam (Ativan) can be useful in treating acute mania and managing the psychomotor agitation often seen in mania.

   ○ Antidepressants – Medications such as bupropion (Wellbutrin) and sertraline (Zoloft) are useful during the depressive phase. These are typically prescribed in combination with a mood stabilizer to prevent rebound mania.

MEDICATION CLASSIFICATION: MOOD STABILIZER

- Select Prototype Medication: lithium carbonate

Purpose

- Expected Pharmacological Action

   ○ Lithium produces neurochemical changes in the brain, including serotonin receptor blockade.

   ○ There is evidence that lithium decreases neuronal atrophy and increases neuronal growth.

- Lithium is used in the treatment of bipolar disorders. Lithium controls episodes of acute mania, helps to prevent the return of mania or depression, and decreases the incidence of suicide.

Complications

- Advise the client that some adverse effects will resolve within a few weeks of starting the medication.

ADVERSE EFFECTS	NURSING INTERVENTIONS/CLIENT EDUCATION
› Gastrointestinal distress (nausea, diarrhea, abdominal pain)	› Advise the client that GI distress is usually transient. › Administer medication with meals or milk.
› Fine hand tremors that can interfere with purposeful motor skills and can be exacerbated by factors such as stress and caffeine	› Administer beta-adrenergic blocking agents such as propranolol (Inderal). › Adjust dosage to be as low as possible, give in divided doses, or use long-acting formulations. › Advise the client to report an increase in tremors, which could be an indication of lithium toxicity.
› Polyuria, mild thirst	› Use a potassium-sparing diuretic, such as spironolactone (Aldactone). › Instruct the client to maintain adequate fluid intake by consuming at least 2 to 3 L of fluid per day from beverages and food sources.
› Weight gain	› Assist the client to follow a healthy diet and regular exercise regimen
› Kidney toxicity	› Monitor the client's I&O. › Adjust dosage, and keep dose at the lowest level necessary. › Check baseline BUN and creatinine, and monitor kidney function periodically.
› Goiter and hypothyroidism with long-term treatment	› Obtain the client's baseline T_3, T_4, and TSH levels prior to starting treatment, and then annually. › Advise the client to monitor for indications of hypothyroidism (cold, dry skin; decreased heart rate, weight gain). › Administer levothyroxine (Synthroid).
› Bradydysrhythmias, hypotension, electrolyte imbalances	› Encourage the client to maintain adequate fluid intake.

LITHIUM TOXICITY		
LITHIUM LEVEL	CLINICAL MANIFESTATIONS	NURSING INTERVENTIONS/CLIENT EDUCATION
Early indications		
Less than 1.5 mEq/L	› Diarrhea, nausea, vomiting, thirst, polyuria, muscle weakness, fine hand tremors, slurred speech	› Instruct the client to withhold the medication, and notify the provider. › Administer new dosage based on the client's serum lithium and sodium levels.
Advanced indications		
1.5 to 2.0 mEq/L	› Mental confusion, poor coordination, coarse tremors, and ongoing GI distress, including nausea, vomiting, and diarrhea	› Instruct the client to withhold the medication, and notify the provider. › Administer new dosage based on the client's serum lithium and sodium levels. › Excretion may need to be promoted.

LITHIUM TOXICITY		
LITHIUM LEVEL	**CLINICAL MANIFESTATIONS**	**NURSING INTERVENTIONS/CLIENT EDUCATION**
Severe toxicity		
Greater than 2.0 to 2.5 mEq/L	› Extreme polyuria of dilute urine, tinnitus, blurred vision, ataxia, seizures, severe hypotension leading to coma, and possible death from respiratory complications	› Administer an emetic to alert clients, or administer gastric lavage. › Assist with clients who are receiving medications to increase the rate of excretion.
Greater than 2.5 mEq/L	› Rapid progression of manifestations leading to coma and death	› Hemodialysis can be warranted.

Contraindications/Precautions

- Lithium is a Pregnancy Risk Category D medication. It is considered teratogenic, especially during the first trimester of pregnancy.
- Discourage clients from breastfeeding if lithium therapy is necessary.
- Use cautiously in clients who have impaired kidney function, heart disease, sodium depletion, and dehydration.

Medication/Food Interactions

MEDICATION/FOOD INTERACTIONS	NURSING INTERVENTIONS/CLIENT EDUCATION
› Diuretics – Sodium is excreted with the use of diuretics. With decreased serum sodium, lithium excretion is decreased, which can lead to toxicity.	› Monitor for indications of toxicity. › Advise the client to observe for indications of toxicity and to notify the provider. › Encourage the client to maintain a diet adequate in sodium, and to drink 2 to 3 L of water a day.
› NSAIDs (ibuprofen [Motrin] and celecoxib [Celebrex]) – Concurrent use will increase renal reabsorption of lithium, leading to toxicity.	› Avoid use of NSAIDs to prevent toxic accumulation of lithium. › Use aspirin as a mild analgesic.
› Anticholinergics (antihistamines, tricyclic antidepressants) – Abdominal discomfort can result from anticholinergic-induced urinary retention and polyuria.	› Advise the client to avoid medications with anticholinergic effects.

Nursing Administration

- Monitor plasma lithium levels while undergoing treatment. At initiation of treatment, monitor levels every 2 to 3 days until stable, and then every 1 to 3 months. Lithium blood levels should be obtained in the morning, usually 12 hr after last dose.

  ○ During initial treatment of a manic episode, levels should be between 0.8 to 1.4 mEq/L.

  ○ Maintenance level range is between 0.4 to 1.0 mEq/L.

  ○ Plasma levels greater than 1.5 mEq/L can result in toxicity.

- Older adult clients are at an increased risk for toxicity and require more frequent monitoring of serum lithium levels.

- Care for a client who has a toxic plasma lithium level should take place in an acute care setting with supportive measures provided. Hemodialysis can be indicated.

- Advise the client that effects begin within 7 to 14 days.

- Advise the client to take lithium as prescribed. This medication must be administered in two or three doses daily due to a short half-life. Taking lithium with food will help decrease GI distress.

- Encourage the client to adhere to laboratory appointments needed to monitor lithium effectiveness and adverse effects. Emphasize the high risk of toxicity due to the narrow therapeutic range.

- Provide nutritional counseling. Stress the importance of adequate fluid and sodium intake.

- Instruct the client to monitor for indications of toxicity and when to contact the provider. The client should withhold the medication and seek medical attention if she is experiencing diarrhea, vomiting, or excessive sweating.

MEDICATION CLASSIFICATION: MOOD-STABILIZING ANTIEPILEPTIC DRUGS (AEDs)

- Select Prototype Medications

  ○ Carbamazepine (Tegretol, Equetro)

  ○ Valproic acid (Depakote)

  ○ Lamotrigine (Lamictal)

Purpose

- Expected Pharmacological Action

  ○ AEDs help treat and manage bipolar disorder through various mechanisms.

    ▪ Slowing the entrance of sodium and calcium back into the neuron, thus extending the time it takes for the nerve to return to its active state

    ▪ Potentiating the inhibitory effects of gamma butyric acid (GABA)

    ▪ Inhibiting glutamic acid (glutamate), which in turn suppresses CNS excitation

- Therapeutic Uses

  ○ These medications are used to treat manic and depressive episodes, as well as to prevent relapse of mania and depressive episodes. They are particularly useful for clients who have mixed mania and rapid cycling bipolar disorders.

Complications

ADVERSE EFFECTS	NURSING INTERVENTIONS/CLIENT EDUCATION
Carbamazepine (Tegretol, Equetro)	
› Minimal effect on cognitive function › CNS effects 　» Nystagmus 　» Double vision 　» Vertigo 　» Staggering gait 　» Headache	› Administer in low doses initially, and then gradually increase dosage. › Advise the client that effects should subside within a few weeks. › Administer dose at bedtime.
› Blood dyscrasias (leukopenia, anemia, thrombocytopenia)	› Obtain baseline CBC and platelets. Perform ongoing monitoring of these. › Observe for indications of thrombocytopenia, including bruising and bleeding of gums. › Monitor for indications of infection, such as fever or lethargy. › Advise the client to notify the provider if indications of blood dyscrasias are present.
› Teratogenesis	› Advise the client to avoid use in pregnancy.
› Hypo-osmolarity – promotes secretion of ADH, which inhibits water excretion by the kidneys, and places the client who has heart failure at risk for fluid overload	› Monitor the client's serum sodium. › Monitor for edema, decrease in urine output, and hypertension.
› Skin disorders, including dermatitis, rash (Stevens-Johnson syndrome)	› Treat mild reactions with anti-inflammatory or antihistamine medications. › Advise the client to wear sunscreen. › Instruct the client to withhold the medication and notify the provider if Stevens-Johnson rash occurs.
Lamotrigine (Lamictal)	
› Double or blurred vision, dizziness, headache, nausea, vomiting	› Caution the client about performing activities that require concentration/visual acuity.
› Serious skin rashes, including Stevens-Johnson syndrome	› Instruct the client to withhold the medication, and notify the provider if a rash occurs.

ADVERSE EFFECTS	NURSING INTERVENTIONS/CLIENT EDUCATION
Valproic Acid (Depakote)	
› GI effects include nausea, vomiting, and indigestion	› Advise the client that these effects are generally self-limiting › Advise the client to take medication with food, or switch to enteric-coated formulations.
› Hepatotoxicity as evidenced by anorexia, nausea, vomiting, fatigue, abdominal pain, jaundice	› Check baseline liver function, and monitor liver function regularly (minimum of every 2 months during the first 6 months of treatment). › Advise the client to observe for indications of hepatotoxicity and to notify the provider immediately if they occur. › Avoid using in children younger than 2 years old. › Administer the lowest effective dose.
› Pancreatitis as evidenced by nausea, vomiting, abdominal pain	› Advise the client to observe for manifestations of pancreatitis and to notify the provider immediately if they occur. › Monitor the client's amylase levels. › Discontinue the medication if pancreatitis develops.
› Thrombocytopenia	› Advise the client to observe for indications, such as bruising, and to notify the provider if these occur. › Monitor the client's platelet counts.
› Teratogenesis	› Advise the client to avoid use during pregnancy. › Advise the client to talk to the provider if she is considering pregnancy to discuss other treatment options.

Contraindications/Precautions

- These medications are Pregnancy Risk Category D medications. They can result in birth defects.
- Carbamazepine is contraindicated in clients who have bone marrow suppression or bleeding disorders.
- Valproic acid is contraindicated in clients who have liver disorders.

Medication/Food Interactions

MEDICATION/FOOD INTERACTIONS	NURSING INTERVENTIONS/CLIENT EDUCATION
Carbamazepine (Tegretol)	
› Oral contraceptives, warfarin (Coumadin) – Concurrent use of carbamazepine causes a decrease in the effects of these medications due to stimulation of hepatic and drug-metabolizing enzymes.	› Advise the client to use an alternate form of birth control. › Monitor for therapeutic effects of warfarin. Dosage can need to be adjusted.
› Grapefruit juice – Inhibits metabolism of carbamazepine, thereby increasing blood levels of the medication.	› Advise the client to avoid all intake of grapefruit juice.
› Phenytoin, phenobarbital – Concurrent use decreases the effects of carbamazepine by stimulating metabolism.	› Monitor phenytoin and phenobarbital levels, and adjust dosages as prescribed.
Lamotrigine (Lamictal)	
› Carbamazepine, phenytoin, phenobarbital – Concurrent use decreases the effect of lamotrigine.	› Monitor for therapeutic effects, and adjust dosages as prescribed.
› Valproic acid – Concurrent use inhibits drug-metabolizing enzymes, thereby increasing the half-life of lamotrigine.	› Monitor for adverse effects, and adjust dosages as prescribed.
› Oral contraceptives – Concurrent use decreases the effectiveness of both medications.	› Advise the client to use an alternate form of birth control.
Valproic Acid (Depakote)	
› Phenytoin, phenobarbital – Serum levels of these medications are increased when used concurrently with valproic acid.	› Monitor phenytoin and phenobarbital levels, and adjust dosages as prescribed.

Nursing Evaluation of Medication Effectiveness

- Depending on therapeutic intent, effectiveness can be evidenced by the following.
  - Relief of acute manic manifestations (flight of ideas, obsessive talking, agitation) or depressive manifestations (fatigue, poor appetite, psychomotor retardation)
  - Verbalization of improvement in mood
  - Ability to perform ADLs
  - Improved sleeping and eating habits
  - Appropriate interaction with peers

APPLICATION EXERCISES

1. A nurse is caring for a client who is on lithium therapy. The client states that he wants to take ibuprofen for osteoarthritis pain relief. Which of the following statements by the nurse is appropriate?

    A. "That is a good choice. Ibuprofen does not interact with lithium."

    B. "Regular aspirin would be a better choice than ibuprofen."

    C. "Lithium decreases the effectiveness of ibuprofen."

    D. "The ibuprofen will make your lithium level fall too low."

2. A nurse is discussing routine follow-up needs for a client who has a new prescription for valproic acid (Depakote). The nurse should inform the client of the need for routine monitoring of which of the following?

    A. AST/ALT and LDH

    B. Creatinine and BUN

    C. WBC and granulocyte counts

    D. Serum sodium and potassium

3. A nurse is discussing early indications of toxicity with a client who has a new prescription for lithium carbonate for bipolar disorder. The nurse should include which of the following when reinforcing teaching? (Select all that apply.)

    _____ A. Constipation

    _____ B. Polyuria

    _____ C. Rash

    _____ D. Muscle weakness

    _____ E. Tinnitus

4. A nurse is caring for a client who is experiencing extreme mania due to bipolar disorder. Prior to administration of lithium carbonate, the nurse notes that the lithium blood level is 1.2 mEq/L. Which of the following is an appropriate action by the nurse?

    A. Administer the next dose of lithium carbonate as scheduled.

    B. Prepare the client for gastric lavage.

    C. Notify the provider for a possible increase in the dosage of lithium carbonate.

    D. Request a stat repeat of the client's lithium blood level.

5. A nurse is assisting with the admission of a client who has a new diagnosis of bipolar disorder and is scheduled to begin lithium therapy. When collecting data about the medical history from the client's adult daughter, which of the following statements is the priority to report to the provider?

   A. "My mother has diabetes that is controlled by her diet."

   B. "My mother recently completed a course of prednisone for acute bronchitis."

   C. "My mother received her flu vaccine last month."

   D. "My mother is currently on furosemide for her congestive heart failure."

6. A nurse is reinforcing teaching to a client who has rapid cycling bipolar disorder and a new prescription for carbamazepine (Equetro). Use the ATI Active Learning Template: Medication to complete this item to include the following sections:

   A. Therapeutic Uses: Discuss the use of carbamazepine as it relates to bipolar disorder.

   B. Adverse Effects: Identify at least four adverse effects.

   C. Nursing Interventions/Client Education: Describe at least four nursing interventions or client education points.

APPLICATION EXERCISES KEY

1. A. INCORRECT: Ibuprofen is not recommended for clients taking lithium.

   B. **CORRECT:** Aspirin is recommended as a mild analgesic, rather than ibuprofen, due to the risk for lithium toxicity.

   C. INCORRECT: Lithium does not decrease the effectiveness of ibuprofen. However, concurrent use is not recommended due to the risk of toxicity.

   D. INCORRECT: Ibuprofen increases the risk for a toxic, rather than low, lithium level.

   (N) NCLEX® Connection: Pharmacological Therapies, Adverse Effects/Contraindications/ Side Effects/Interactions

2. A. **CORRECT:** Routine monitoring of liver function tests is necessary due to the risk for hepatotoxicity.

   B. INCORRECT: Baseline levels may be drawn. However, routine monitoring of creatinine and BUN is not necessary.

   C. INCORRECT: Baseline levels may be drawn. However, routine monitoring of WBC and granulocyte counts is not necessary.

   D. INCORRECT: Baseline levels may be drawn. However, routine monitoring of serum sodium and potassium is not necessary.

   (N) NCLEX® Connection: Pharmacological Therapies, Medication Administration

3. A. INCORRECT: Diarrhea, rather than constipation, is an early indication of lithium toxicity.

   B. **CORRECT:** Polyuria is an early indication of lithium toxicity.

   C. INCORRECT: A rash is not indication of lithium toxicity.

   D. **CORRECT:** Muscle weakness is an early indication of lithium toxicity.

   E. INCORRECT: Tinnitus is an indication of severe, rather than early, toxicity.

   (N) NCLEX® Connection: Pharmacological Therapies, Adverse Effects/Contraindications/ Side Effects/Interactions

4. A. **CORRECT:** During a manic episode, the lithium blood level should be between 0.8 to 1.4 mEq/L. Therefore, it is appropriate to administer the next dose as scheduled.

   B. INCORRECT: Gastric lavage may be prescribed for treatment of severe toxicity for levels between 2.0 to 2.5 mEq/L.

   C. INCORRECT: A dosage increase would place the client at risk for toxicity and is therefore not an appropriate action.

   D. INCORRECT: A lithium level of 1.2 mEq/L is an expected finding for a client who is experiencing a manic episode. Therefore, it is not necessary to request a stat repeat of the laboratory test.

   (N) NCLEX® Connection: Pharmacological Therapies, Medication Administration

5. A. INCORRECT: It is important to notify the provider of the client's medical history. However, this information does not pose the greatest risk to the client and is therefore not the priority.

    B. INCORRECT: It is important to notify the provider of the client's medical history. However, this information does not pose the greatest risk to the client and is therefore not the priority.

    C. INCORRECT: It is important to notify the provider of the client's medical history. However, this information does not pose the greatest risk to the client and is therefore not the priority.

    D. **CORRECT:** Diuretics, such as furosemide (Lasix), are contraindicated for use with lithium due to the risk for toxicity. This is the greatest risk for the client and is therefore the priority to report to the provider.

    N NCLEX® Connection: Pharmacological Therapies, Adverse Effects/Contraindications/Side Effects/ Interactions

6. *Using ATI Active Learning Template: Medication*

    A. Therapeutic Uses
    - Carbamazepine is used to treat manic and depressive episodes, as well as to prevent relapse of mania and depressive episodes of bipolar disorder. This type of medication is particularly useful for clients who have mixed mania and rapid cycling bipolar disorders.

    B. Adverse Effects
    - CNS effects
      ○ Nystagmus
      ○ Diplopia
      ○ Vertigo
      ○ Staggering gait
      ○ Headache
    - Blood dyscrasias
    - Teratogenesis
    - Hypo-osmolarity
    - Dermatitis
    - Rash

    C. Nursing Interventions/Client Education
    - Advise the client that CNS effects should subside within a few weeks.
    - Administer carbamazepine at bedtime to minimize CNS effects.
    - Advise the client of the need for routine monitoring of CBC, platelets, and serum sodium levels.
    - Monitor for indications of bleeding.
    - Advise the client to avoid use in pregnancy.
    - Monitor the client for indications of fluid retention.
    - Advise the client to wear sunscreen.
    - Instruct the client to notify the provider if a rash occurs.

    N NCLEX® Connection: Pharmacological Therapies, Expected Actions/Outcomes

chapter 22

Overview

- Schizophrenia spectrum disorders are the primary reason for the administration of antipsychotic medications.

  ○ The clinical course of schizophrenia usually involves acute exacerbations with intervals of semiremission in which manifestations remain present but are less severe.

  ○ Medications are used to treat:

    ▪ Positive symptoms related to behavior, thought, and speech (agitation, delusions, hallucinations, tangential speech patterns).

    ▪ Negative symptoms (social withdrawal, lack of emotion, lack of energy, flattened affect, decreased motivation, decreased pleasure in activities).

- The goals of psychopharmacological treatment for schizophrenia spectrum and other psychotic disorders include the following.

  ○ Suppression of acute episodes

  ○ Prevention of acute recurrence

  ○ Maintenance of the highest possible level of functioning

- First-generation (conventional) antipsychotic medications are used mainly to control positive symptoms of psychotic disorders and are reserved for clients who are:

  ○ Using them successfully and can tolerate the adverse effects.

  ○ Violent or particularly aggressive.

- Second-generation (atypical) antipsychotic agents are the current medications of choice for clients receiving initial treatment, and for treating breakthrough episodes in clients on conventional medication therapy, because they are more effective with fewer adverse effects.

  ○ Advantages of atypical antipsychotic agents

    ▪ Relief of both positive and negative symptoms.

    ▪ Decrease in affective findings (depression, anxiety) and suicidal behaviors.

    ▪ Improvement of neurocognitive deficits, such as poor memory.

    ▪ Fewer or no extrapyramidal symptoms (EPS), including tardive dyskinesia, due to less dopamine blockade.

    ▪ Fewer anticholinergic effects, with the exception of clozapine (Clozaril), which has a high incidence of anticholinergic effects. This is because most of the atypical antipsychotics cause little or no blockade of cholinergic receptors.

    ▪ Less relapse.

MEDICATION CLASSIFICATION:
ANTIPSYCHOTICS FIRST-GENERATION (CONVENTIONAL)

- Select Prototype Medication: chlorpromazine, low potency
- Other Medications
  - Haloperidol (Haldol), high potency
  - Fluphenazine, high potency
  - Loxapine, medium potency
  - Thioridazine, low potency
  - Thiothixene (Navane), high potency
  - Perphenazine, medium potency
  - Trifluoperazine, high potency

Purpose

- Expected Pharmacological Action
  - The conventional antipsychotic medications block dopamine (D2), acetylcholine, histamine, and norepinephrine (NE) receptors in the brain and periphery.
  - Inhibition of psychotic manifestations is believed to be a result of D2 blockade in the brain.
- Therapeutic Uses
  - Acute and chronic psychotic disorders
  - Schizophrenia spectrum disorders
  - Bipolar disorder – primarily the manic phase
  - Tourette's disorder
  - Prevention of nausea/vomiting through blocking of dopamine in the chemoreceptor trigger zone of the medulla

Complications

AGRANULOCYTOSIS	
Nursing Interventions/ Client Education	› Advise clients to observe for indications of infection (fever, sore throat), and to notify the provider if these occur. › If indications of infection appear, obtain baseline WBC. Medication should be discontinued if laboratory test indicates the presence of infection.

ANTICHOLINERGIC EFFECTS		
Manifestations	› Dry mouth › Blurred vision	› Photophobia › Urinary hesitancy or retention	› Constipation › Tachycardia
Nursing Interventions/ Client Education	› Suggest the following strategies to decrease anticholinergic effects. » Chewing sugarless gum » Sipping on water » Avoiding hazardous activities » Wearing sunglasses when outdoors	» Eating foods high in fiber » Participating in regular exercise » Maintaining fluid intake of 2 to 3 L/day from beverages and food sources » Voiding just before taking medication	

EXTRAPYRAMIDAL SYMPTOMS (EPS)	
ACUTE DYSTONIA	
Manifestations	› Severe spasm of the tongue, neck, face, and back › Crisis situation that requires rapid treatment
Nursing Interventions/ Client Education	› Begin to monitor for acute dystonia anywhere between 5 hr to 5 days after administration of first dose. › Treat with anticholinergic agents, such as benztropine (Cogentin) or diphenhydramine.
PARKINSONISM	
Manifestations	› Bradykinesia › Shuffling gait › Tremors › Rigidity › Drooling
Nursing Interventions/ Client Education	› Observe for parkinsonism for the first month after the initiation of therapy. › Treat with benztropine, diphenhydramine, or amantadine (Symmetrel).
AKATHISIA	
Manifestations	› Inability to sit or stand still › Continual pacing and agitation
Nursing Interventions/ Client Education	› Observe for akathisia for the first 2 months after the initiation of treatment. › Manage with beta-blockers, benzodiazepines, or anticholinergic medications.
TARDIVE DYSKINESIA (TD)	
Manifestations	› Late EPS › Involuntary movements of the tongue and face, such as lip smacking and tongue fasciculations › Involuntary movements of the arms, legs, and trunk
Nursing Interventions/ Client Education	› Administer lowest dosage possible to control manifestations. › Evaluate the client after 12 months of therapy and then every 3 months. Manifestations can occur months to years after the initiation of therapy. If TD appears, dosage should be lowered, or the client should be switched to an atypical agent.

NEUROENDOCRINE EFFECTS	
Manifestations	› Gynecomastia › Galactorrhea › Menstrual irregularities
Nursing Interventions/ Client Education	› Advise the client to observe for these manifestations and to notify the provider if they occur.

NEUROLEPTIC MALIGNANT SYNDROME	
Manifestations	› Sudden high fever › Dysrhythmias › Muscle rigidity › Blood pressure fluctuations › Changes in level of consciousness › Coma
Nursing Interventions/ Client Education	› Most commonly occurs within the first 2 weeks of treatment. › Apply cooling blankets. › Stop antipsychotic medication. › Increase the client's fluid intake. › Monitor vital signs. › Wait 2 weeks before resuming therapy. Consider switching to an atypical agent. › Administer antipyretics, such as aspirin or acetaminophen.

ORTHOSTATIC HYPOTENSION	
Nursing Interventions/ Client Education	› The client should develop tolerance in 2 to 3 months. › Monitor blood pressure and heart rate for orthostatic changes. Hold medication until the provider is notified of significant changes. › Instruct clients about the indications of postural hypotension (lightheadedness, dizziness). If these occur, advise the client to sit or lie down. Orthostatic hypotension can be minimized by getting up or changing positions slowly.

SEDATION	
Nursing Interventions/ Client Education	› Inform the client that effects should diminish within a few weeks. › Instruct the client to take the medication at bedtime to avoid daytime sleepiness. › Advise the client not to drive until sedation has subsided.

SEIZURES	
Indications	› Greatest risk in clients who have an existing seizure disorder
Nursing Interventions/ Client Education	› Advise the client to report seizure activity to the provider. › An increase in antiseizure medication may be necessary.

SEVERE DYSRHYTHMIAS	
Nursing Interventions/ Client Education	› Obtain baseline ECG and potassium level prior to treatment, and periodically throughout the treatment period. › Avoid concurrent use with other medications that prolong QT interval.

SEXUAL DYSFUNCTION	
Note	› Common in both males and females
Nursing Interventions/ Client Education	› Advise the client of possible adverse effects. › Encourage the client to report effects to the provider. › The client can need dosage lowered or be switched to a high-potency agent.

SKIN EFFECTS	
Manifestations	› Photosensitivity that can result in severe sunburn › Contact dermatitis from handling medications
Nursing Interventions/ Client Education	› Advise clients to avoid excessive exposure to sunlight, to use sunscreen, and to wear protective clothing. › Advise clients to avoid direct contact with the medication.

Contraindications/Precautions

- These medications are contraindicated in clients who are in a coma, or who have severe depression, Parkinson's disease, prolactin-dependent cancer of the breast, or severe hypotension.

- Use of conventional antipsychotic medications is contraindicated in older adult clients who have dementia.

- Use cautiously in clients who have glaucoma, paralytic ileus, prostate enlargement, heart disorders, liver or kidney disease, and seizure disorders.

Medication/Food Interactions

MEDICATION/FOOD INTERACTIONS	NURSING INTERVENTIONS/CLIENT EDUCATION
› Anticholinergic agents – Concurrent use with other anticholinergic medications will increase effects.	› Advise the client to avoid over-the-counter medications that contain anticholinergic agents, such as sleep aids.
› CNS depressants – Additive CNS depressant effects with concurrent use of alcohol, opioids, and antihistamines.	› Advise the client to avoid alcohol and other medications that cause CNS depression. › Advise the client to avoid hazardous activities, such as driving.
› Levodopa – By activating dopamine receptors, levodopa counteracts effects of antipsychotic agents.	› Advise the client to avoid concurrent use of levodopa and other direct dopamine receptor agonists.

Nursing Administration

- Use the Abnormal Involuntary Movement Scale (AIMS) to screen for the presence of EPS.
- Monitor the client to differentiate between EPS and worsening of a psychotic disorder.
- Administer anticholinergics, beta-blockers, and benzodiazepines to control early EPS. If symptoms are intolerable, a client can be switched to a low-potency or atypical antipsychotic agent.
- Advise clients that antipsychotic medications do not cause addiction.
- Advise clients to take medication as prescribed and on a regular schedule.
- Advise clients that some therapeutic effects can be noticeable within a few days, but significant improvement can take 2 to 4 weeks, and possibly several months for full effects.

- Consider depot preparations, administered IM once every 2 to 4 weeks, for clients who have difficulty maintaining a medication regimen. Inform the client that lower doses can be used with depot preparations, which will decrease the risk of adverse effects and the development of tardive dyskinesia.
- Begin administration with twice-daily dosing, but switch to daily dosing at bedtime to decrease daytime drowsiness and promote sleep.

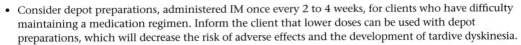

MEDICATION CLASSIFICATION:
ANTIPSYCHOTICS SECOND-GENERATION (ATYPICAL)

- Select Prototype Medication: risperidone (Risperdal)
- Other Medications
  - Aripiprazole (Abilify)
  - Asenapine (Saphris)
  - Clozapine (Clozaril)
  - Iloperidone (Fanapt)
  - Lurasidone (Latuda)
  - Olanzapine (Zyprexa)
  - Paliperidone (Invega)
  - Quetiapine (Seroquel)
  - Ziprasidone (Geodon)

Purpose

- Expected Pharmacological Action
  - These antipsychotic agents work mainly by blocking serotonin, and to a lesser degree, dopamine receptors. These medications also block receptors for norepinephrine, histamine, and acetylcholine.
- Therapeutic Uses
  - Negative and positive symptoms of schizophrenia spectrum disorders
  - Psychosis induced by levodopa therapy
  - Relief of psychotic manifestations in other disorders, such as bipolar disorder

Complications

ADVERSE EFFECTS	NURSING INTERVENTIONS/CLIENT EDUCATION
› New onset of diabetes mellitus or loss of glucose control in clients who have diabetes	› Obtain baseline fasting blood glucose, and monitor the value periodically throughout treatment. › Instruct the client to report indications, such as increased thirst, urination, and appetite, to the provider.
› Weight gain	› Advise the client to follow a healthy, low-calorie diet, engage in regular exercise, and monitor weight gain.
› Hypercholesterolemia with increased risk for hypertension and other cardiovascular disease	› Monitor cholesterol, triglycerides, and blood glucose if weight gain is greater than 14 kg (30 lb).
› Orthostatic hypotension	› Monitor blood pressure and heart rate for orthostatic changes. › Hold medication while notifying the provider of significant changes.
› Anticholinergic effects, such as urinary hesitancy or retention, dry mouth	› Monitor for these adverse effects, and report their occurrence to the provider. › Encourage the client to use measures to relieve dry mouth, such as sipping water throughout the day.
› Agitation, dizziness, sedation, and sleep disruption	› Monitor for these adverse effects, and report their occurrence to the provider. › Administer an alternative medication if prescribed.
› Mild EPS, such as tremor	› Monitor for and reinforce teaching to clients on how to recognize EPS. › Use AIMS test to screen for EPS.

Contraindications/Precautions

- Risperidone
    - Risperidone is a Pregnancy Risk Category C medication.
    - These medications should not be used for clients who have dementia. Use of these medications can cause death related to cerebrovascular accident or infection.
    - Clients should avoid the concurrent use of alcohol.
    - Use cautiously in clients who have cardiovascular or cerebrovascular disease, seizures, or diabetes mellitus. Clients who have diabetes mellitus should have a baseline fasting blood sugar, and blood glucose should be monitored carefully.

- Other Atypical Antipsychotic Agents

MEDICATION	FORMULATIONS	COMMENTS
Aripiprazole (Abilify)	› Tablets › Orally disintegrating tablets › Oral solution › Short-acting injectable	› Low or no risk of EPS › Low or no risk of diabetes, weight gain, dyslipidemia, orthostatic hypotension, and anticholinergic effects › Adverse effects » Sedation » Headache » Anxiety » Insomnia » Gastrointestinal upset
Asenapine (Saphris)	› Sublingual tablets	› Low risk of diabetes, weight gain, dyslipidemia, and anticholinergic effects › Other adverse effects » Drowsiness » Prolonged QT interval » EPS (higher doses) » Temporary numbing of the mouth
Clozapine (Clozaril) – The first atypical antipsychotic developed, it is no longer considered a first-line medication for schizophrenia spectrum disorders due to its adverse effects.	› Tablets › Orally disintegrating tablets	› Low risk of EPS › High risk of weight gain, diabetes, and dyslipidemia › Risk for fatal agranulocytosis » Baseline and weekly monitoring of WBC recommended » Notify the provider of indications of infection (fever, sore throat, mouth lesions) › Other adverse effects » Sedation » Orthostatic hypotension » Anticholinergic effects
Iloperidone (Fanapt)	› Tablets	› Significant risk for weight gain, prolonged QT interval, and orthostatic hypotension » Advise clients to follow titration schedule during initial therapy to minimize hypotension. › Low risk for diabetes, dyslipidemia, and EPS › Common adverse effects » Dry mouth » Sedation » Fatigue » Nasal congestion

MEDICATION	FORMULATIONS	COMMENTS
Lurasidone (Latuda)	› Tablets	› Low risk for diabetes, weight gain, and dyslipidemia. › Does not cause anticholinergic effects › Common adverse effects » Sedation » Akathisia » Parkinsonism » Agitation and anxiety » Nausea
Olanzapine (Zyprexa)	› Tablets › Short-acting injectable › Extended-release injection	› Low risk of EPS › High risk of diabetes, weight gain, and dyslipidemia › Other adverse effects » Sedation » Orthostatic hypotension » Anticholinergic effects
Paliperidone (Invega, Invega Sustenna)	› Extended-release tablets › Extended-release injections	› Significant risk for diabetes, weight gain, and dyslipidemia › Other adverse effects » Sedation » Prolonged QT interval » Orthostatic hypotension » Anticholinergic effects » Mild EPS
Quetiapine (Seroquel)	› Tablets › Extended-release tablets	› Low risk of EPS › Moderate risk of diabetes, weight gain, and dyslipidemia › Other adverse effects » Cataracts » Sedation » Orthostatic hypotension » Anticholinergic effects
Ziprasidone (Geodon) – This medication affects both dopamine and serotonin, so it can be used for clients who have concurrent depression.	› Capsules › Short-acting injectable	› Low risk of EPS › Low risk of diabetes, weight gain, and dyslipidemia › Other adverse effects » Sedation » Orthostatic hypotension » Anticholinergic effects » ECG changes and QT prolongation that can lead to *torsades de pointes*

Medication/Food Interactions

MEDICATION/FOOD INTERACTIONS	NURSING INTERVENTIONS/CLIENT EDUCATION
› Immunosuppressive medications, such as anticancer medications, can further suppress immune function.	› Avoid use in clients who are taking clozapine.
› Additive CNS depressant effects can occur with concurrent use of alcohol, opioids, antihistamines, and other CNS depressants.	› Advise clients to avoid alcohol and other medications that cause CNS depression. › Advise clients to avoid hazardous activities, such as driving.
› Levodopa – By activating dopamine receptors, levodopa counteracts the effects of antipsychotic agents.	› Avoid concurrent use of levodopa and other direct dopamine receptor agonists.
› Tricyclic antidepressants, amiodarone (Cordarone), and clarithromycin (Biaxin) prolong QT intervals, thereby increasing the risk of cardiac dysrhythmias.	› Atypical antipsychotics that prolong the QT interval should not be used concurrently with other medications that have the same effect.
› Barbiturates and phenytoin (Dilantin) stimulate hepatic drug-metabolizing enzymes, thereby decreasing drug levels of aripiprazole, quetiapine, and ziprasidone.	› Monitor medication effectiveness.
› Fluconazole (Diflucan) inhibits hepatic drug-metabolizing enzymes, thereby increasing drug levels of aripiprazole, quetiapine, and ziprasidone.	› Monitor medication effectiveness.

Nursing Administration

- Risperidone also is available as a depot injection administered IM once every 2 weeks. This method of administration is a good option for clients who have difficulty adhering to a medication schedule. Therapeutic effect occurs 4 to 6 weeks after first depot injection.
- Advise clients that low doses of medication are given initially, and dosages are then gradually increased.
- Use oral disintegrating tablets for clients who may attempt to "cheek" or "pocket" tablets, or for those who have difficulty swallowing them.
- Advise clients taking asenapine to avoid eating or drinking for 10 min after each dose.
- Administer lurasidone with food to increase absorption.

- The cost of antipsychotic medications can be a factor for some clients. Evaluate the need for case management intervention.

Nursing Evaluation of Medication Effectiveness

- Depending on therapeutic intent, effectiveness can be evidenced by:
  - ○ Improvement and/or prevention of acute psychotic manifestations, absence of hallucinations, delusions, anxiety, hostility.
  - ○ Improvement in ability to perform ADLs.
  - ○ Improvement in ability to interact socially with peers.
  - ○ Improvement of sleeping and eating habits.

APPLICATION EXERCISES

1. A nurse is caring for a client who has schizophrenia and exhibits a lack of grooming and a flat affect. The nurse should anticipate a prescription of which of the following medications?

    A. Chlorpromazine

    B. Thiothixene (Navane)

    C. Risperidone (Risperdal)

    D. Haloperidol (Haldol)

2. A nurse is caring for a client who takes ziprasidone (Geodon). The client reports difficulty swallowing the oral medication and becomes extremely agitated with injectable administration. The nurse should contact the provider to discuss a change to which of the following medications? (Select all that apply.)

    _____ A. Olanzapine (Zyprexa)

    _____ B. Quetiapine (Seroquel)

    _____ C. Aripiprazole (Abilify)

    _____ D. Clozapine (Clozaril)

    _____ E. Paliperidone (Invega)

3. A nurse is discussing manifestations of schizophrenia with a newly licensed nurse. Which of the following should the nurse identify as being effectively treated by conventional antipsychotics? (Select all that apply.)

    _____ A. Auditory hallucinations

    _____ B. Withdrawal from social situations

    _____ C. Delusions of grandeur

    _____ D. Severe agitation

    _____ E. Anhedonia

4. A nurse is collecting data on a client who is currently taking perphenazine. Which of the following findings should the nurse identify as an extrapyramidal symptom (EPS)? (Select all that apply.)

    _____ A. Decreased level of consciousness

    _____ B. Drooling

    _____ C. Involuntary arm movements

    _____ D. Urinary retention

    _____ E. Continual pacing

5. A nurse is reinforcing discharge teaching with a client who has schizophrenia and a new prescription for iloperidone (Fanapt). Which of the following client statements indicates understanding of the teaching?

    A. "I will be able to stop taking this medication as soon as I feel better."

    B. "If I feel drowsy during the day, I will stop taking this medication and call my provider."

    C. "I will be careful not to gain too much weight while taking this medication."

    D. "This medication is highly addictive and must be withdrawn slowly."

6. A nurse is reinforcing teaching to a client who has a new prescription for clozapine (Clozaril). Use the ATI Active Learning Template: Medication to complete this item to include the following sections:

    A. Therapeutic Uses: Identify two.

    B. Adverse Effects: Identify at least four.

    C. Evaluation of Medication Effectiveness: Identify at least two outcomes.

APPLICATION EXERCISES KEY

1. A. INCORRECT: Conventional antipsychotics, such as chlorpromazine, are used mainly to control positive, rather than negative, symptoms of schizophrenia.

   B. INCORRECT: Conventional antipsychotics, such as thiothixene, are used mainly to control positive, rather than negative, symptoms of schizophrenia.

   C. **CORRECT:** Atypical antipsychotics, such as risperidone, are effective in treating negative symptoms of schizophrenia, such as lack of grooming and flat affect.

   D. INCORRECT: Conventional antipsychotics, such as haloperidol, are used mainly to control positive, rather than negative, symptoms of schizophrenia.

   Ⓝ NCLEX® Connection: Pharmacological Therapies, Expected Actions/Outcomes

2. A. INCORRECT: Olanzapine is available only in tablet or injectable form and will therefore not address the current concerns with medication administration.

   B. INCORRECT: Quetiapine is available only in tablets or extended-release tablets and will therefore not address the current concerns with medication administration.

   C. **CORRECT:** Aripiprazole is available in an orally disintegrating tablet, which is appropriate for clients who have difficulty swallowing oral tablets. This route also decreases the risk for agitation associated with an injection.

   D. **CORRECT:** Clozapine is available in an orally disintegrating tablet, which is appropriate for clients who have difficulty swallowing oral tablets. This route also decreases the risk for agitation associated with an injection.

   E. INCORRECT: Paliperidone is available only in extended-release tablets or injections and will therefore not address the current concerns with medication administration.

   Ⓝ NCLEX® Connection: Pharmacological Therapies, Adverse Effects/Contraindications/ Side Effects/Interactions

3. A. **CORRECT:** Positive symptoms of schizophrenia, such as auditory hallucinations, are effectively treated with conventional antipsychotics.

   B. INCORRECT: Conventional antipsychotics have minimal effectiveness with negative symptoms of schizophrenia, such as social withdrawal.

   C. **CORRECT:** Positive symptoms of schizophrenia, such as delusions of grandeur, are effectively treated with conventional antipsychotics.

   D. **CORRECT:** Positive symptoms of schizophrenia, such as severe agitation, are effectively treated with conventional antipsychotics.

   E. INCORRECT: Conventional antipsychotics have minimal effectiveness with negative symptoms of schizophrenia, such as anhedonia.

   Ⓝ NCLEX® Connection: Pharmacological Therapies, Expected Actions/Outcomes

4. A. INCORRECT: Decreased level of consciousness is an indication of neuroleptic malignant syndrome, rather than an EPS.

    B. **CORRECT:** Drooling is an indication of parkinsonism, which is an EPS.

    C. **CORRECT:** Involuntary arm movements are an indication of tardive dyskinesia, which is an EPS.

    D. INCORRECT: Urinary retention is an anticholinergic effect rather than an EPS.

    E. **CORRECT:** Continual pacing is an indication of akathisia, which is an EPS.

    Ⓝ NCLEX® Connection: Pharmacological Therapies, Adverse Effects/Contraindications/ Side Effects/Interactions

5. A. INCORRECT: Antipsychotic medications are considered a long-term treatment for schizophrenia. Discontinuing the medication can result in an exacerbation of manifestations.

    B. INCORRECT: Drowsiness is a common adverse effect of antipsychotic medications. However, it is not appropriate to discontinue the medication.

    C. **CORRECT:** Antipsychotic medications, such as iloperidone, have a high risk for significant weight gain.

    D. INCORRECT: Antipsychotic medications are not considered addictive, and it is not necessary to titrate iloperidone when discontinuing treatment.

    Ⓝ NCLEX® Connection: Pharmacological Therapies, Adverse Effects/Contraindications/ Side Effects/Interactions

6. *Using the ATI Active Learning Template: Medication*

    A. Therapeutic Uses
    - Treatment of negative and positive symptoms of schizophrenia spectrum disorders
    - Psychosis induced by levodopa therapy
    - Relief of psychotic manifestations in nonpsychotic disorders, such as bipolar disorder

    B. Adverse Effects
    - Weight gain
    - Diabetes mellitus
    - Dyslipidemia
    - Agranulocytosis
    - Sedation
    - Orthostatic hypotension
    - Anticholinergic effects

    C. Evaluation of Medication Effectiveness
    - Improvement of positive and negative symptoms
    - Improvement in ability to perform ADLs
    - Improvement in ability to interact socially with peers
    - Improvement in sleeping and eating habits

    Ⓝ NCLEX® Connection: Pharmacological Therapies, Expected Actions/Outcomes

chapter 23

Overview

- Various medications are used to manage behavioral disorders in children and adolescents. Parents should understand that pharmacological management is most effective when accompanied by techniques to modify behavior.

- Medications include tricyclic antidepressants, antipsychotics, nonbarbiturate anxiolytics, CNS stimulants, and norepinephrine selective reuptake inhibitors.

MEDICATION CLASSIFICATION: CNS STIMULANTS

MEDICATION	SHORT-ACTING	INTERMEDIATE-ACTING	LONG-ACTING
Methylphenidate	› Ritalin, Methylin	› Ritalin SR, Methylin ER	› Ritalin LA, Concerta, Daytrana (transdermal)
Dexmethylphenidate	› Focalin		› Focalin XR
Dextroamphetamine	› Dexedrine		› Dexedrine spansules
Amphetamine Mixture	› Adderall		› Adderall XR
Lisdexamfetamine dimesylate			› Vyvanse

Purpose

- Expected Pharmacological Action
  - These medications raise the levels of norepinephrine, serotonin, and dopamine into the central nervous system.
- Therapeutic Uses
  - ADHD in children and adults
  - Conduct disorder

Complications

ADVERSE EFFECTS	NURSING INTERVENTIONS/CLIENT EDUCATION
› CNS stimulation (insomnia, restlessness)	› Advise the client to observe for effects, and to notify the provider if they occur. › Decrease dosage as prescribed. › Administer the last dose of the day before 4 p.m.
› Weight loss	› Monitor the client's weight and compare to baseline height and weight. › Administer medication right before or after meals. › Encourage children to eat at regular meal times and to avoid unhealthy food choices.
› Cardiovascular effects (dysrhythmias, chest pain, high blood pressure) – can increase the risk of sudden death in clients who have heart abnormalities	› Monitor vital signs and ECG. › Advise clients to observe for effects and to notify the provider if they occur.
› Development of psychotic manifestations, such as hallucinations, paranoia	› Instruct the client to report manifestations immediately and discontinue the medication.
› Withdrawal reaction	› Advise the client to avoid abrupt cessation of the medication, as it could lead to depression and severe fatigue.
› Hypersensitivity skin reaction to transdermal methylphenidate – hives, papules	› Advise the client to remove the patch and notify the provider.

Contraindications/Precautions

- Contraindicated in clients who have a history of substance use disorder, cardiovascular disorders, severe anxiety, and psychosis.

Medication/Food Interactions

MEDICATION/FOOD INTERACTIONS	NURSING INTERVENTIONS/CLIENT EDUCATION
› MAOIs – concurrent use can cause hypertensive crisis.	› Avoid concurrent use.
› Caffeine – concurrent use can cause an increase in CNS stimulant effects.	› Instruct the client to avoid foods and beverages that contain caffeine.
› Phenytoin (Dilantin), warfarin (Coumadin), and phenobarbital – methylphenidate inhibits metabolism of these medications, leading to increased serum levels.	› Monitor for adverse effects (CNS depression, signs of bleeding). › Concurrent use of these medications is done with caution.
› OTC cold and decongestant medications – concurrent use can lead to increased CNS stimulation.	› Instruct the client to avoid the use of these OTC medications.

Nursing Administration

- Advise clients to swallow sustained-release tablets whole and to not chew or crush them.

- Explain to the client the importance of administering the medication on a regular schedule.

- Instruct clients who use transdermal medication (Daytrana) to place the patch on one hip daily in the morning, and leave it in place no longer than 9 hr. Alternate hips daily.

 - Instruct parents and clients that ADHD is not cured by the medication. Management in conjunction with an overall treatment plan that includes family and cognitive therapy will improve outcomes.

- Instruct parents that these medications have special handling procedures controlled by federal law. Handwritten prescriptions are required for medication refills.

- Instruct parents regarding safety and storage of medications.

- Advise parents that these medications have a high potential for development of a substance use disorder, especially in adolescents.

Nursing Evaluation of Medication Effectiveness

- Depending on therapeutic intent, effectiveness can be evidenced by improvement of manifestations of ADHD, such as an increased ability to focus and complete tasks, interact with peers, and manage impulsivity.

MEDICATION CLASSIFICATION: NOREPINEPHRINE SELECTIVE REUPTAKE INHIBITOR

- Select Prototype Medication: atomoxetine (Strattera)

Purpose

- Expected Pharmacological Action

  ○ Block reuptake of norepinephrine at synapses in the CNS. Atomoxetine is not a stimulant medication.

- Therapeutic Uses

  ○ ADHD in children and adults

Complications

ADVERSE EFFECTS	NURSING INTERVENTIONS/CLIENT EDUCATION
Usually tolerated well with minimal side effects	
› Appetite suppression, weight loss, growth suppression	› Monitor the client's weight and compare to baseline height and weight. › Administer medication right before meals. › Encourage children to eat at regular meal times and avoid unhealthy food choices.
› GI effects (nausea, vomiting)	› Advise the client to take the medication with food if GI effects occur.
› Suicidal ideation (in children and adolescents)	› Monitor for indications of depression. › Advise the client to report changes in mood, excessive sleeping, agitation, irritability.
› Hepatotoxicity	› Advise the client to report indications of liver damage, such as flulike manifestations, yellowing skin, and abdominal pain.

Contraindications/Precautions

- Use cautiously in clients who have cardiovascular disorders.

Medication/Food Interactions

MEDICATION/FOOD INTERACTIONS	NURSING INTERVENTIONS/CLIENT EDUCATION
› MAOIs – concurrent use can cause hypertensive crisis.	› Advise the client to avoid concurrent use.
› Paroxetine (Paxil), fluoxetine (Prozac), and quinidine gluconate (Quinidine) inhibit metabolizing enzymes, thereby increasing levels of atomoxetine.	› Instruct the client to watch for and report increased adverse effects of atomoxetine. › Concurrent use can require a reduction in the dosage of atomoxetine.

Nursing Administration

- Note any changes in the client related to dosing and timing of medications.
- Administer the medication in one daily dose in the morning or in two divided doses, morning and afternoon, with or without food.
- Instruct the client that therapeutic effect can take 1 to 3 weeks to fully develop.

Nursing Evaluation of Medication Effectiveness

- Depending on therapeutic intent, effectiveness can be evidenced by improvement of the manifestations of ADHD, such as increase in ability to focus, complete tasks, interact with peers, and manage impulsivity.

MEDICATION CLASSIFICATION: TRICYCLIC ANTIDEPRESSANTS (TCAs)

- Select Prototype Medication: desipramine (Norpramin)
- Other Medications
  - Imipramine (Tofranil)
  - Clomipramine (Anafranil)

Purpose

- Expected Pharmacological Action
  - These medications block reuptake of the monoamine neurotransmitters norepinephrine and serotonin in the synaptic space, thereby intensifying their effects.
- Therapeutic Uses in Children
  - Depression
  - Autism spectrum disorder
  - ADHD
  - Panic, school phobia, separation anxiety disorder
  - OCD

Complications

ADVERSE EFFECTS	NURSING INTERVENTIONS/CLIENT EDUCATION
› Orthostatic hypotension	› Monitor blood pressure with first dose. › If orthostatic hypotension occurs, instruct the client to change positions slowly.
› Anticholinergic effects » Dry mouth » Blurred vision » Photophobia » Urinary hesitancy or retention » Constipation » Tachycardia	› Instruct the client regarding ways to minimize anticholinergic effects. » Chewing gum » Sipping water » Avoiding hazardous activities » Wearing sunglasses when outdoors » Eating foods high in fiber » Participating in regular exercise » Increasing fluid intake to at least 2 to 3 L/day from beverages and other food sources » Voiding just before taking the medication › Advise the client to notify the provider if effects become intolerable.
› Weight gain	› Monitor the client's weight. › Encourage the client to participate in regular exercise and to follow a healthy, low-calorie diet.

ADVERSE EFFECTS	NURSING INTERVENTIONS/CLIENT EDUCATION
› Sedation	› Advise the client that sedative effects should diminish over time › Advise the client to avoid hazardous activities, such as driving if sedation is excessive. › Advise the client to take the medication at bedtime to minimize daytime sleepiness and to promote sleep.
› Toxicity resulting in cholinergic blockade and cardiac toxicity evidenced by dysrhythmias, mental confusion, and agitation followed by seizures and coma	› Give a client who is acutely ill a 1-week supply of medication. › Obtain baseline ECG. › Monitor vital signs frequently. › Monitor toxicity. › Notify the provider if indications of toxicity occur.
› Decreased seizure threshold	› Monitor clients who have seizure disorders.
› Excessive sweating	› Inform the client of this adverse effect, and assist with frequent linen changes.

Contraindications/Precautions

- Use cautiously in clients who have seizure disorders; diabetes; liver, kidney and respiratory disorders; and hyperthyroidism.

Medication/Food Interactions

MEDICATION/FOOD INTERACTIONS	NURSING INTERVENTIONS/CLIENT EDUCATION
› MAOIs – concurrent use causes hypertension.	› Do not administer concurrently with MAOIs.
› Antihistamines and other anticholinergic agents – concurrent use can cause additive anticholinergic effects.	› Do not administer concurrently with antihistamines.
› Epinephrine and dopamine (direct-acting sympathomimetics) – concurrent use can cause hypertensive effect.	› Do not administer these medications concurrently with TCAs.
› Alcohol, benzodiazepines, opioids, and antihistamines – concurrent use can cause additive CNS depression.	› Advise the client to avoid other CNS depressants while taking a TCA.

Nursing Administration

- Instruct the client's parents to administer this medication as prescribed on a daily basis to establish therapeutic plasma levels.

- Assist with the client's medication regimen adherence by informing the client and parents that it can take 1 to 3 weeks to experience therapeutic effects. Full therapeutic effects can take 2 to 3 months.

- Instruct the client and parents on the importance of continuing therapy after improvement in manifestations. Sudden discontinuation of the medication can result in relapse.

- Give only a 1-week supply of medication for a client who is acutely ill, and then only give a 1-month supply of medication at a time.

Nursing Evaluation of Medication Effectiveness

- Effectiveness for clients who have depression can be evidenced by:
  - Verbalization of improvement in mood.
  - Improved sleeping and eating habits.
  - Increased interaction with peers.
- Effectiveness for clients who have autism spectrum disorder can be evidenced by:
  - Decreased anger.
  - Decreased compulsive behavior.
- Effectiveness for clients who have ADHD can be evidenced by:
  - Decreased hyperactivity.
  - Greater ability to pay attention.

MEDICATION CLASSIFICATION: ALPHA$_2$-ADRENERGIC AGONISTS

- Select Prototype Medication: guanfacine (Intuniv)
- Other Medication: clonidine (Kapvay)

Purpose

- Expected Pharmacological Action
  - The action of alpha$_2$-adrenergic agonists is not completely understood. However, they are known to activate presynaptic alpha$_2$-adrenergic receptors within the brain.
- Therapeutic Use
  - ADHD

Complications

ADVERSE EFFECTS	NURSING INTERVENTIONS/CLIENT EDUCATION
› CNS effects (sedation, drowsiness, fatigue)	› Monitor for these adverse effects, and report their occurrence to the provider. › Advise the client to avoid hazardous activities
› Cardiovascular effects (hypotension, bradycardia)	› Monitor blood pressure and pulse, especially during initial treatment. › Advise the client not to abruptly discontinue medication, which can cause rebound hypertension.
› Weight gain	› Monitor weight. › Encourage the client to participate in regular exercise and to follow a healthy, well-balanced diet.

Contraindications/Precautions

- Extended-release clonidine is contraindicated for children less than 6 years old.
- Use cautiously in clients who have cardiac disease.

Interactions

MEDICATION/FOOD INTERACTIONS	NURSING INTERVENTIONS/CLIENT EDUCATION
› CNS depressants, including alcohol, can increase CNS effects.	› Avoid concurrent use.
› Antihypertensives can worsen hypotension.	› Avoid concurrent use.
› Foods with high-fat content increase guanfacine absorption.	› Advise the client to avoid taking medication with a high-fat meal.

Nursing Administration

- Monitor for the use of alcohol and CNS depressants, especially with adolescent clients.
- Instruct clients to not chew, crush, or split extended-release preparations.
- Monitor blood pressure and pulse at baseline, with initial treatment, and with each dosage change.
- Advise clients to avoid abrupt discontinuation of medication, which can result in rebound hypertension. Medication should be tapered according to a prescribed dosage schedule when discontinuing treatment.

Nursing Evaluation of Medication Effectiveness

- Depending on therapeutic intent, effectiveness can be evidenced by improvement of manifestations of ADHD, such as increase in ability to focus, complete tasks, interact with peers, and manage impulsivity.

MEDICATION CLASSIFICATION: ANTIPSYCHOTICS-ATYPICAL

- Select Prototype Medication: risperidone (Risperdal)
- Other Medication: olanzapine (Zyprexa)

Purpose

- Expected Pharmacological Action
  - These antipsychotic agents work mainly by blocking serotonin, and to a lesser degree, dopamine receptors. These medications also block receptors for norepinephrine, histamine, and acetylcholine.
- Therapeutic Uses
  - Pervasive development disorders (PDD), including autism spectrum disorder
  - Conduct disorder
  - PTSD
  - Relief of psychotic manifestations

Complications

ADVERSE EFFECTS	NURSING INTERVENTIONS/CLIENT EDUCATION
› New onset of diabetes mellitus or loss of glucose control in clients who have diabetes	› Obtain baseline fasting blood glucose, and monitor periodically throughout treatment. › Instruct the client to report indications such as increased thirst, urination, and appetite.
› Weight gain	› Advise the client to follow a healthy low-calorie diet, engage in regular exercise, and monitor weight gain.
› Hypercholesterolemia with increased risk for hypertension and other cardiovascular disease	› Monitor cholesterol, triglycerides, and blood glucose if weight gain is more than 14 kg (31 lb).
› Orthostatic hypotension	› Monitor blood pressure with first dose, and instruct the client to change positions slowly if orthostatic hypotension occurs.
› Anticholinergic effects (urinary retention or hesitancy, dry mouth)	› Monitor for these adverse effects, and report their occurrence to the provider. › Encourage client to use measures to relieve dry mouth, such as sipping fluids throughout the day.
› Symptoms of agitation, dizziness, sedation, and sleep disruption	› Monitor for these adverse effects, and report their occurrence to the provider. › Administer an alternative medication if prescribed.
› Mild extrapyramidal symptoms (EPSs), such as tremor	› Monitor for and teach clients to recognize EPSs. These effects are usually dose-related.

Contraindications/Precautions

- Be aware of possible alcohol use in the adolescent client. Instruct clients to avoid the use of alcohol.
- Use cautiously in clients who have cardiovascular disease, seizures, or diabetes. Clients who have diabetes should have a baseline fasting blood sugar, and blood glucose should be monitored carefully.

MEDICATION/FOOD INTERACTIONS	NURSING INTERVENTIONS/CLIENT EDUCATION
› CNS depressants – additive CNS depression occurs with concurrent use of alcohol, opioids, antihistamines.	› Advise the client to avoid alcohol and other medications that cause CNS depression. › Advise the client to avoid hazardous activities, such as driving.
› Levodopa – by activating dopamine receptors, levodopa counteracts the effects of antipsychotic agents.	› Avoid concurrent use of levodopa and other direct dopamine receptor agonists.
› Tricyclic antidepressants amiodarone (Cordarone), and clarithromycin (Biaxin) prolong QT interval, thereby increasing the risk of cardiac dysrhythmias.	› Avoid concurrent use of these medications.
› Barbiturates and phenytoin (Dilantin) promote hepatic drug-metabolizing enzymes, thereby decreasing drug levels of quetiapine.	› Monitor medication for effectiveness.
› Fluconazole (Diflucan) inhibits hepatic drug-metabolizing enzymes, thereby increasing drug levels of aripiprazole, quetiapine, and ziprasidone.	› Monitor for adverse medication effects.

Nursing Administration

- Administer by oral or IM route.
  - Risperidone is available in an oral solution and quick-dissolving tablets for ease in administration.
  - Olanzapine is available in an orally disintegrating tablet for ease in administration.
- Advise clients that low doses of medication are given initially and are then gradually increased.

Nursing Evaluation of Medication Effectiveness

- Effectiveness for clients who have PDD is evidenced by:
  - Reduction of hyperactivity.
  - Improvement in mood.
- Effectiveness for clients who have conduct disorder is evidenced by decreased aggressiveness.
- Effectiveness for clients who have PTSD is evidenced by:
  - Decreased aggressiveness and reduction of flashbacks.
  - Improvement of psychosis (prevention of acute psychotic manifestations, absence of hallucinations, delusions, anxiety, hostility).
  - Improvement in ability to perform ADLs.
  - Improvement in ability to interact socially with peers.
  - Improvement of sleeping and eating habits.

APPLICATION EXERCISES

1. A nurse is reinforcing teaching with the parents of a child who has a new prescription for imipramine (Tofranil) about possible indications of toxicity. Which of the following would be appropriate for the nurse to include? (Select all that apply.)

_____ A. Seizures

_____ B. Agitation

_____ C. Photophobia

_____ D. Dry mouth

_____ E. Irregular pulse

2. A nurse is reinforcing teaching with an adolescent client who has OCD and a new prescription for clomipramine (Anafranil). Which of the following instructions should the nurse include to minimize one of the adverse effects of his medication?

A. Eat a diet high in fiber.

B. Check temperature daily.

C. Take medication first thing in the morning before eating.

D. Add extra calories to the diet as between-meal snacks.

3. A nurse is reinforcing teaching with an adolescent who is to begin taking atomoxetine (Strattera) for ADHD. The nurse should instruct the client to monitor for and report which of the following indications of liver damage? (Select all that apply).

_____ A. Mood changes

_____ B. Yellowing skin

_____ C. Joint pain

_____ D. Fever

_____ E. Malaise

4. A nurse is caring for a school-age child who has a new prescription for methylphenidate (Daytrana) to treat ADHD. Which of the following should the nurse instruct the client and family about this medication?

    A. Apply the patch once daily at bedtime.

    B. Take the medication orally with food every 12 hr.

    C. Take a second dose of the medication orally at bedtime.

    D. Remove the patch each day after 9 hr.

5. A nurse is reinforcing teaching with a school-age child and his parents about a new prescription for lisdexamfetamine dimesylate (Vyvanse). Which of the following is appropriate for the nurse to include in the instructions? (Select all that apply).

    _____ A. An adverse effect of this medication is CNS depression.

    _____ B. Administer the medication right before breakfast.

    _____ C. Monitor blood pressure while taking this medication.

    _____ D. Therapeutic effects of this medication will take 1 to 3 weeks to fully develop.

    _____ E. This medication blocks the effects of dopamine in the brain.

6. A nurse working in a pediatric mental health clinic is caring for a client who has a new prescription for olanzapine (Zyprexa) for the treatment of PTSD. Use the Medication ATI Active Learning Template to complete this item to include the following sections:

    A. Side/Adverse Effects: Identify at least four adverse effects of this medication.

    B. Nursing Interventions/Client Education: Identify at least four nursing interventions to prevent or minimize the adverse effects of this medication.

APPLICATION EXERCISES KEY

1. A. **CORRECT:** Seizures are an indication of TCA toxicity.

    B. **CORRECT:** Agitation is an indication of TCA toxicity.

    C. INCORRECT: Photophobia is an anticholinergic effect rather than an indication of TCA toxicity.

    D. INCORRECT: Dry mouth is an anticholinergic effect rather than an indication of TCA toxicity.

    E. **CORRECT:** Irregular pulse can indicate a dysrhythmia, which is an indication of TCA toxicity.

    Ⓝ NCLEX® Connection: Pharmacological Therapies, Adverse Effects/Contraindications/
    Side Effects/Interactions

2. A. **CORRECT:** Eating a diet high in fiber will decrease constipation, which is an anticholinergic effect associated with TCA use.

    B. INCORRECT: Checking the client's temperature daily is not necessary while taking a TCA.

    C. INCORRECT: Taking the medication at bedtime rather than in the morning is appropriate to prevent daytime sleepiness.

    D. INCORRECT: Following a well-balanced diet plan rather than adding extra calories as snacks will help prevent weight gain, a common adverse effect of TCAs.

    Ⓝ NCLEX® Connection: Pharmacological Therapies, Adverse Effects/Contraindications/
    Side Effects/Interactions

3. A. INCORRECT: Mood changes are a possible of indication of depression rather than hepatotoxicity.

    B. **CORRECT:** Yellowing skin is a potential indication of hepatotoxicity that the client should report to the provider.

    C. INCORRECT: Abdominal, rather than joint, pain is a potential indication of hepatotoxicity that the client should report to the provider.

    D. **CORRECT:** Fever is a potential indication of hepatotoxicity that the client should report to the provider.

    E. **CORRECT:** Malaise is a potential indication of hepatotoxicity that the client should report to the provider.

    Ⓝ NCLEX® Connection: Pharmacological Therapies, Adverse Effects/Contraindications/
    Side Effects/Interactions

4. A. INCORRECT: Daytrana is a transdermal patch that is applied once daily in the morning.

    B. INCORRECT: Oral preparations of methylphenidate are available. However, Daytrana is a transdermal patch.

    C. INCORRECT: Oral preparations of methylphenidate are available. However, Daytrana is a transdermal patch.

    D. **CORRECT:** Daytrana is a transdermal patch that is applied once daily in the morning and is removed after 9 hr.

    Ⓝ NCLEX® Connection: Pharmacological Therapies, Medication Administration

5. A. INCORRECT: An adverse effect of Vyvanse is CNS stimulation rather than CNS depression.

    B. **CORRECT:** Administer Vyvanse immediately before or after a meal due to appetite suppression.

    C. **CORRECT:** Monitoring blood pressure is appropriate due to potential cardiovascular effects of Vyvanse.

    D. INCORRECT: Atomoxetine (Strattera), rather than Vyvanse, takes 1 to 3 weeks to fully develop therapeutic effects.

    E. INCORRECT: Vyvanse, a CNS stimulant, works by raising the levels of norepinephrine, serotonin, and dopamine into the CNS.

    Ⓝ NCLEX® Connection: Pharmacological Therapies, Medication Administration

6. *Using the Medication ATI Active Learning Template*

    A. Side/Adverse Effects

    - New onset of diabetes mellitus or loss of glucose control in clients who have diabetes
    - Weight gain
    - Hypercholesterolemia
    - Orthostatic hypotension
    - Anticholinergic effects (urinary hesitancy or retention, dry mouth)
    - Agitation
    - Dizziness
    - Sedation
    - Sleep disruption
    - Tremors

    B. Nursing Interventions/Client Education

    - Obtain fasting blood glucose prior to and periodically throughout treatment.
    - Instruct the client to report indications of diabetes mellitus, including increased thirst, urination, and appetite.
    - Advise clients to follow a healthy, well-balanced diet.
    - Recommend regular exercise.
    - Monitor weight throughout treatment.
    - Monitor cholesterol and triglycerides, especially if weight gain is more than 30 lb.
    - Monitor blood pressure with first dose and instruct client to change positions slowly.
    - Encourage the client to sip fluids throughout the day.

    Ⓝ NCLEX® Connection: Pharmacological Therapies, Adverse Effects/Contraindications/ Side Effects/Interactions

chapter 24

Overview

- Abstinence syndrome occurs when a client abruptly withdraws from a drug on which he is physically dependent.
- Withdrawing from a substance that has the potential to cause abstinence syndrome can cause distressing manifestations that also can be life-threatening.

WITHDRAWAL MANIFESTATIONS FOR MAJOR SUBSTANCES ASSOCIATED WITH SUBSTANCE USE DISORDER
Alcohol
› Manifestations usually start within 4 to 12 hr of the last intake of alcohol, peak after 24 to 48 hr, and then suddenly disappear, unless alcohol withdrawal delirium occurs.
› Common manifestations include nausea; vomiting; tremors; restlessness and inability to sleep; depressed mood or irritability; increased heart rate, blood pressure, respiratory rate, and temperature; and tonic-clonic seizures. Illusions are also common.
› Alcohol withdrawal delirium can occur 2 to 3 days after cessation of alcohol and can last 2 to 3 days. This is considered a medical emergency. Manifestations include severe disorientation, psychotic effects (hallucinations), severe hypertension, cardiac dysrhythmias, and delirium. This type of withdrawal can progress to death.
Opioids
› Withdrawal manifestations occur within hours to several days after cessation of opioid use.
› Common findings include agitation, insomnia, flulike manifestations, rhinorrhea, yawning, sweating, and diarrhea.
› Withdrawal manifestations are not life-threatening, although suicidal ideation can occur.
Tobacco (nicotine)
› Abstinence syndrome is evidenced by irritability, nervousness, restlessness, insomnia, and difficulty concentrating.

- Other substances associated with substance use disorder include cannabis, hallucinogens, inhalants, sedatives/hypnotics, and stimulants.

MEDICATIONS TO SUPPORT WITHDRAWAL/ABSTINENCE FROM ALCOHOL

Detoxification

BENZODIAZEPINES	
Examples	› Chlordiazepoxide (Librium) › Diazepam (Valium) › Lorazepam (Ativan) › Oxazepam
Intended Effects	› Maintenance of vital signs within the expected reference range › Decrease in the risk of seizures › Decrease in the intensity of withdrawal manifestations
Nursing Interventions/ Client Education	› Administer around the clock or PRN. › Obtain baseline vital signs. › Monitor vital signs and neurological status on an ongoing basis. › Provide for seizure precautions (padded side rails, suction equipment at bedside).

ADJUNCT MEDICATIONS	
Examples	› Carbamazepine (Tegretol) › Clonidine (Catapres) › Propranolol (Inderal)
Intended Effects	› Decrease in seizures – carbamazepine › Depression of autonomic response (decrease in blood pressure, heart rate) – clonidine and propranolol › Decrease in craving – propranolol
Nursing Interventions/ Client Education	› Provide for seizure precautions (padded side rails, suction equipment at bedside). › Obtain baseline vital signs, and continue to monitor on an ongoing basis.

Abstinence Maintenance (Following Detoxification)

DISULFIRAM (ANTABUSE)	
Intended Effects	› Disulfiram is a daily oral medication that is a type of aversion (behavioral) therapy. › Disulfiram used concurrently with alcohol will cause acetaldehyde syndrome to occur. » Effects include nausea, vomiting, weakness, sweating, palpitations, and hypotension. › Acetaldehyde syndrome can progress to respiratory depression, cardiovascular suppression, seizures, and death.
Nursing Interventions/ Client Education	› Inform the client of the potential dangers of drinking any alcohol. › Advise the client to avoid any products that contain alcohol (cough syrups, aftershave lotion). › Encourage the client to wear a medical alert bracelet. › Encourage the client to participate in a 12-step program. › Advise the client that medication effects, such as the potential for acetaldehyde syndrome with alcohol ingestion, persist for 2 weeks following discontinuation of disulfiram. › Monitor liver function tests to detect hepatotoxicity.

NALTREXONE (VIVITROL)	
Intended Effects	› Naltrexone is a pure opioid antagonist that suppresses the craving and pleasurable effects of alcohol (also used for opioid withdrawal).
Nursing Interventions/ Client Education	› Collect data about the client's history to determine whether the client is also dependent on opioids. Concurrent use increases the risk for overdose of opiates. › Advise the client to take naltrexone with meals to decrease gastrointestinal distress. › Suggest monthly IM injections for clients who have difficulty adhering to the medication regimen.

ACAMPROSATE (CAMPRAL)	
Intended Effects	› Acamprosate is taken orally three times a day to reduce the craving for alcohol.
Nursing Interventions/ Client Education	› Inform the client that diarrhea can result. Advise the client to maintain adequate fluid intake to prevent dehydration. › Advise the client to avoid use in pregnancy.

MEDICATIONS TO SUPPORT WITHDRAWAL/ABSTINENCE FROM OPIOIDS

METHADONE (DOLOPHINE) SUBSTITUTION

Intended Effects	› Methadone substitution is an oral opioid agonist that replaces the opioid to which the client is addicted. › Methadone administration prevents abstinence syndrome from occurring and removes the need for the client to obtain illegal opioids. › Methadone substitution is used for withdrawal and long-term maintenance. › Dependence is transferred from the illegal opioid to methadone.
Nursing Interventions/ Client Education	› Encourage the client to participate in a 12-step program. › Inform the client that the medication must be administered from an approved treatment center.

CLONIDINE (CATAPRES)

Intended Effects	› Clonidine assists with withdrawal effects related to autonomic hyperactivity (diarrhea, nausea, vomiting). › Clonidine therapy does not reduce the craving for opioids.
Nursing Interventions/ Client Education	› Obtain baseline vital signs. › Advise the client to avoid activities that require mental alertness until drowsiness subsides. › Encourage the client to chew gum or suck on hard candy, and to sip on small amounts of water or suck on ice chips to treat dry mouth.

BUPRENORPHINE (SUBOXONE)

Intended Effects	› Buprenorphine is an agonist-antagonist opioid used for both detoxification and maintenance. › This medication decreases feelings of craving and can be effective in maintaining compliance.
Nursing Interventions/ Client Education	› Inform the client that the medication must be administered from an approved treatment center. › Administer the medication sublingually.

MEDICATIONS TO SUPPORT WITHDRAWAL/ABSTINENCE FROM NICOTINE

BUPROPION (ZYBAN)

Intended Effects	› Bupropion decreases nicotine craving and manifestations of withdrawal.
Nursing Interventions/ Client Education	› To treat dry mouth, encourage the client to chew sugarless gum, suck on hard candy, sip on small amounts of water, or suck on ice chips. › Advise the client to avoid caffeine and other CNS stimulants to control insomnia.

NICOTINE REPLACEMENT THERAPY (NICOTINE GUM [NICORETTE], NICOTINE PATCH [NICOTROL], NICOTINE NASAL SPRAY [NICOTROL NS])

Intended Effects	› Nicotine replacements are pharmaceutical product substitutes for the nicotine in cigarettes or chewing tobacco. › The rate of tobacco use cessation is nearly doubled with the use of nicotine replacements.
Nursing Interventions/ Client Education	› Use of nicotine gum is not recommended for longer than 6 months. › Advise the client to » Chew gum slowly and intermittently over 30 min. » Avoid eating or drinking 15 min prior to and while chewing the gum. » Apply a nicotine patch to an area of clean, dry skin each day. » Avoid using any nicotine products while wearing the patch. » Remove the patch and notify the provider if a local skin reaction occurs. » Remove the patch prior to magnetic resonance imaging (MRI). » Nasal spray provides pleasurable effects of smoking due to rapid rise of nicotine in the blood level. » One spray in each nostril delivers the amount of nicotine in one cigarette. » Advise client to follow product instructions for dosage of nasal spray frequency. » Nicotine nasal spray is not recommended for clients who have disorders affecting the upper respiratory system such as chronic sinus problems, allergies, or asthma. » Avoid using any nicotine products while pregnant or breastfeeding.

VARENICLINE (CHANTIX)	
Intended Effects	› Varenicline is a nicotinic receptor agonist that promotes the release of dopamine to simulate the pleasurable effects of nicotine. › Reduces cravings for nicotine as well as the severity of withdrawal manifestations. › Reduces the incidence of relapse by blocking the desired effects of nicotine.
Nursing Interventions/ Client Education	› Instruct client to take medication after a meal. › Monitor blood pressure during treatment. › Monitor clients who have diabetes mellitus for loss of glycemic control. › Follow instructions for titration to minimize adverse effects. › Advise client to notify the provider if nausea, vomiting, insomnia, new-onset depression, or suicidal thoughts occur. › Contraindicated for clients who have chronic depression, serious mental illness, or suicidal ideation.

Nursing Evaluation of Medication Effectiveness

- Depending on therapeutic intent, effectiveness can be evidenced by:
    - Absence of injury.
    - Ongoing abstinence from the substance.
    - Regular attendance at a 12-step program.

APPLICATION EXERCISES

1. A nurse is reinforcing teaching to a client who has alcohol use disorder and a new prescription for carbamazepine (Tegretol). Which of the following should the nurse include in the teaching?

    A. "This medication will help prevent seizures during alcohol withdrawal."

    B. "Taking this medication will decrease your cravings for alcohol."

    C. "This medication maintains your blood pressure at a normal level during alcohol withdrawal."

    D. "Taking this medication will improve your ability to maintain abstinence from alcohol."

2. A nurse is assisting in the discharge planning for a client following alcohol detoxification. The nurse should anticipate prescriptions for which of the following medications to promote long-term abstinence from alcohol? (Select all that apply.)

    _____ A. Lorazepam (Ativan)

    _____ B. Diazepam (Valium)

    _____ C. Disulfiram (Antabuse)

    _____ D. Naltrexone (Vivitrol)

    _____ E. Acamprosate (Campral)

3. A nurse is caring for a client who has an opioid use disorder and is evaluating the client's understanding of a new prescription for clonidine (Catapres). Which of the following statements by the client indicates an understanding of the teaching?

    A. "Taking this medication will help reduce my craving for heroin."

    B. "While taking this medication, I should keep a pack of sugarless gum."

    C. "I can expect some diarrhea because of taking this medicine."

    D. "Each dose of this medication should be placed under my tongue to dissolve."

4. A nurse is reinforcing teaching with a client who has tobacco use disorder about the use of nicotine gum (Nicorette). Which of the following is appropriate to include in the teaching?

    A. Chew the gum for no more than 10 min.

    B. Rinse out the mouth immediately before chewing the gum.

    C. Avoid eating 15 min prior to chewing the gum.

    D. Use of the gum is limited to 90 days.

5. A nurse is discussing the use of methadone (Dolophine) with a newly licensed nurse. Which of the following statements by the newly licensed nurse indicates a need for further teaching?

    A. "Methadone is a replacement for the client's opioid addiction."

    B. "Methadone reduces the unpleasant effects associated with abstinence syndrome."

    C. "Methadone can be used during opioid withdrawal and to maintain abstinence."

    D. "Methadone increases the client's risk for acetaldehyde syndrome."

6. A nurse working in an outpatient clinic is reinforcing teaching with a client who has tobacco use disorder about the use of varenicline (Chantix). Use the ATI Active Learning Template: Medication to complete this item to include the following sections:

    A. Expected Pharmacological Action

    B. Therapeutic Use

    C. Nursing Interventions/Client Education: Identify at least three.

APPLICATION EXERCISES KEY

1. A. **CORRECT:** Carbamazepine is used during detoxification to decrease the risk for seizures.

    B. INCORRECT: Carbamazepine is used to promote safe detoxification rather than to decrease cravings for alcohol.

    C. INCORRECT: Clonidine or propranolol, rather than carbamazepine, is used during detoxification to depress the autonomic response and its effect on blood pressure.

    D. INCORRECT: Carbamazepine is used to promote safe detoxification rather than abstinence.

    (N) NCLEX® Connection: Pharmacological Therapies, Expected Actions/Outcomes

2. A. INCORRECT: Lorazepam is prescribed for short-term use during detoxification.

    B. INCORRECT: Diazepam is prescribed for short-term use during detoxification.

    C. **CORRECT:** Disulfiram promotes abstinence through aversion therapy.

    D. **CORRECT:** Naltrexone promotes abstinence by suppressing the craving and pleasurable effects of alcohol.

    E. **CORRECT:** Acamprosate decreases the unpleasant effects resulting from abstinence.

    (N) NCLEX® Connection: Pharmacological Therapies, Expected Actions/Outcomes

3. A. INCORRECT: Clonidine is useful during opioid withdrawal. However, it does not reduce cravings.

    B. **CORRECT:** Clonidine commonly causes clients to experience dry mouth. Chewing gum is an effective method to address this adverse effect.

    C. INCORRECT: Clonidine reduces, rather than causes, diarrhea and other withdrawal manifestations related to autonomic hyperactivity.

    D. INCORRECT: Buprenorphine, rather than clonidine, is administered sublingually.

    (N) NCLEX® Connection: Pharmacological Therapies, Adverse Effects/Contraindications/ Side Effects/Interactions

4. A. INCORRECT: The client should chew the gum slowly and intermittently over 30 min.

    B. INCORRECT: The client should avoid drinking 15 min prior to chewing the gum.

    C. **CORRECT:** It is appropriate for the client to avoid eating or drinking 15 min prior to and while chewing the gum.

    D. INCORRECT: Use of nicotine gum is not recommended for longer than 6 months.

    (N) NCLEX® Connection: Pharmacological Therapies, Medication Administration

5. A. INCORRECT: Methadone substitution is an oral opioid agonist that replaces the opioid to which the client is addicted.

    B. INCORRECT: Methadone administration prevents abstinence syndrome from occurring.

    C. INCORRECT: Methadone substitution is used for both opioid withdrawal and long-term maintenance.

    D. **CORRECT:** Disulfiram, rather than methadone, places the client at risk for acetaldehyde syndrome if the client consumes alcohol while taking the medication.

    (N) NCLEX® Connection: Pharmacological Therapies, Medication Administration

6. *Using the ATI Active Learning Template: Medication*

    A. Expected Pharmacological Action
       - Varenicline is a nicotinic receptor agonist that promotes the release of dopamine to simulate the pleasurable effects of nicotine.

    B. Therapeutic Use
       - Varenicline is used to reduce cravings for nicotine as well as the severity of withdrawal manifestations. Varenicline also reduces the incidence of relapse by blocking the desired effects of nicotine.

    C. Nursing Interventions/Client Education
       - Instruct the client to take medication after a meal.
       - Monitor blood pressure during treatment.
       - Monitor for indications of diabetes mellitus.
       - Monitor clients who have diabetes mellitus for loss of glycemic control.
       - Advise the client to follow instructions for titration to minimize adverse effects.
       - Advise the client to notify the provider if nausea, vomiting, insomnia, new-onset depression, or suicidal thoughts occur.
       - Collect data for indications or history of chronic depression, serious mental illness, or suicidal ideation.

    (N) NCLEX® Connection: Pharmacological Therapies, Medication Administration

UNIT 5   ## Special Populations

CHAPTERS

› Care of Those Who Are Dying and/or Grieving
› Mental Health Issues of Children and Adolescents

NCLEX® CONNECTIONS

When reviewing the chapters in this unit, keep in mind the relevant sections of the NCLEX® outline, in particular:

Client Needs: Psychosocial Integrity

› Relevant topics/tasks include:
  » End-of-Life Concepts
    › Identify the client's ability to cope with end-of-life interventions.
  » Grief and Loss
    › Identify the client's reaction to loss (denial, fear).
    › Provide the client with resources to adjust to loss and bereavement (individual counseling, support groups).
  » Mental Health Concepts
    › Assist in the care of a client experiencing sensory or perceptual alterations.
    › Explore why the client is refusing or not following the treatment plan.

chapter 25

Overview

- Clients experience loss in many aspects of their lives.

- Grief is the inner emotional response to loss and is exhibited in as many ways as there are individuals.

- Bereavement includes both grief and mourning (the outward display of loss) as a person deals with the death of a significant individual.

- Palliative, or end-of-life, care is an important aspect of nursing care that attempts to meet the client's physical and psychosocial needs.

- End-of-life issues include decision-making in a highly stressful time during which the nurse must consider the desires of the client and the family. Any decisions must be shared with other health care personnel for a smooth transition during this time of stress, grief, and bereavement.

- Advance directives – Legal documents that direct end-of-life issues.

    ○ Living wills – Directive documents that give specific instructions for medical treatment per a client's wishes.

    ○ Durable power of attorney for health care – A document that appoints an individual to make medical decisions when a client is no longer able to do so on his own behalf.

TYPES OF LOSS	
Necessary loss	› Part of the cycle of life, anticipated but can still be intensely felt
Actual loss	› Any loss of a valued person or item
Perceived loss	› Any loss defined by a client that is not obvious to others
Maturational loss	› Losses normally expected due to the developmental processing of life
Situational loss	› Unanticipated loss caused by an external event

Theories of Grief

- Kübler-Ross: Five Stages of Grief – Stages might not be experienced in order, and the length of each stage will vary from person to person.
  - Denial – The client has difficulty believing a terminal diagnosis or loss.
  - Anger – Anger is directed toward self, others, or objects.
  - Bargaining – The client negotiates for more time or a cure.
  - Depression – The client mourns and directly confronts feelings related to the loss.
  - Acceptance – The client accepts what is happening and plans for the future.
- Worden: Four Tasks of Mourning – Completion of all four tasks generally takes about a year, but this can also vary from person to person.
  - Task I – Accepting the reality of the loss.
  - Task II – Using coping mechanisms to experience the emotional pain of the loss.
  - Task III – Changing the environment to accommodate the absence of the deceased.
  - Task IV – Finding a meaningful connection with the lost entity while learning to live again.

Factors Influencing Loss, Grief, and Coping Ability

- An individual's current stage of development
- Interpersonal relationships and social support network
- Type and significance of the loss
- Culture and ethnicity
- Spiritual and religious beliefs and practices
- Prior experience with loss
- Socioeconomic status
- Dysfunctional grieving risks
  - Being dependent upon the deceased
  - Unexpected death at a young age, through violence, or by a socially unacceptable manner
  - Inadequate coping skills or lack of social support
  - Pre-existing mental health issues, such as depression or substance use disorder

Data Collection

TYPES OF GRIEF	
Normal grief	› This grief is considered uncomplicated. › Emotions can include anger, resentment, withdrawal, hopelessness, and guilt but should change to acceptance with time. › Some acceptance should be evident by 6 months after the loss. › Somatic complaints can include chest pain, palpitations, headaches, nausea, changes in sleep patterns, or fatigue.
Anticipatory grief	› This grief implies the "letting go" of an object or person before the loss, as in the case of a terminal illness. › Individuals have the opportunity to grieve before the actual loss.
Dysfunctional grief	› This grief involves difficult progression through the expected stages of the grieving process. › Usually the work of grief is prolonged, the clinical manifestations are more severe, and they can result in depression or exacerbation of a pre-existing disorder. › The client can develop suicidal ideation, intense feelings of guilt, and lowered self-esteem. › Somatic complaints persist for an extended period of time.
Disenfranchised grief	› This grief entails an experienced loss that cannot be publicly shared or is not socially acceptable, such as the loss of a loved one through suicide.
Grief experienced by public tragedy	› This type of grief is a loss shared by a community or group of individuals. It can include terrorist attacks, assassinations, natural disasters, work or school shootings.

Nursing Interventions

- Facilitate Mourning
  - Grant time for the grieving process.
  - Identify expected grieving behaviors, such as crying, somatic manifestations, and anxiety.
  - Use therapeutic communication. Name the emotion that the client is feeling. For example, a nurse can say, "You sound as though you are angry. Anger is a normal feeling for someone who has lost a loved one. Tell me about how you are feeling."
  - Avoid communication that inhibits open expression of feelings, such as offering false reassurance, giving advice, changing the subject, and taking the focus away from the individual who is grieving.
  - When relating to someone who is bereaved, avoid cliches such as, "She is in a better place now." Rather, encourage the individual to share memories about the decreased.
  - Assist the individual to accept the reality of the loss.
  - Support the client's efforts to "move on" in the face of the loss.
  - Encourage the building of new relationships.
  - Provide continuing support. Encourage the support of family and friends.

○ Check for signs of ineffective coping, such as refusing to leave home months after a client's spouse has died.

○ Share information about mourning and grieving with the client, who might not realize that feelings, such as anger toward the deceased, are expected.

○ Encourage the client who is grieving to attend a bereavement or grief support group.

○ Discuss referral for psychotherapy for a client who is having difficulty resolving grief with the charge nurse.

○ Provide information on available community resources.

○ Ask the client if contacting a spiritual adviser would be acceptable, or encourage the client to do so.

○ Participate in debriefing provided by professional grief/mental health counselors.

 View Video: Caring for Those Who are Grieving or Dying

PALLIATIVE CARE

Overview

- The nurse serves as an advocate for a client's sense of dignity and self-esteem by providing palliative care at the end of life.

- Palliative care improves the quality of life of clients and their families facing end-of-life issues.

- As dementia is a leading cause of death among older adults, nurses must consider the unique aspects of palliative dementia care.

- Palliative care interventions are used primarily when caring for clients who are dying and family members who are grieving.

- Palliative care can be provided by an interprofessional team of providers, nurses, social workers, physical and occupational therapists, spiritual care providers, nutritionists, and pharmacists.

- Hospice care is a comprehensive care delivery system for the terminally ill that is usually implemented when a client is not expected to live longer than 6 months. Further medical care aimed toward a cure is discontinued, and the focus becomes symptom relief and maintaining the client's quality of life. Maintaining quality requires an intentional focus on the physical, social, psychological, and spiritual needs of clients and their families.

Assessment

CHARACTERISTICS OF DISCOMFORT	
› Pain	› Dehydration
› Anxiety	› Diarrhea or constipation
› Dyspnea	› Urinary incontinence
› Nausea or vomiting	› Inability to perform ADLs

CLINICAL FINDINGS OF APPROACHING DEATH	
› Decreased level of consciousness	› Nonreactive pupils
› Muscle relaxation	› Weak pulse and dropping blood pressure
› Altered breathing (labored or irregular, apnea, Cheyne-Stokes pattern)	› Cool extremities
	› Perspiration
› Mucus collection in large airways	› Decreased urine output
› Incontinence of bowel and/or bladder	› Inability to swallow
› Occurrence of mottling with poor circulation	

- Determine the client's sources of strength and hope.
- Identify the desires and expectations of the family and client for end-of-life care.

Nursing Interventions

- Promote continuity of care and communication by limiting assigned staff changes.
- Assist the client and family to set priorities for end-of-life care.
- Physical Care
  - Give priority to the control of symptoms.
  - Administer medications that manage pain, air, hunger, and anxiety.
  - Perform ongoing data collection to determine effectiveness of treatment and need for modifications of treatment plan, such as lower or higher doses of medications.
  - Manage side effects of medications.
  - Reposition the client to maintain airway and comfort.
  - Maintain integrity of skin and mucous membranes.
  - Provide an environment that promotes dignity and self-esteem.
    - Remove products of elimination as soon as possible to maintain a clean and odor-free environment.
    - Offer comfortable clothing.
    - Provide grooming for hair, nails, and skin.
    - Encourage family members to bring in comforting possessions to make the client feel at home.
  - Encourage use of relaxation techniques, such as guided imagery and music.
  - Promote decision-making in food selection, activities, and health care to permit the client as much control as possible.
  - Encourage the client to perform ADLs if the ability and desire exist.

- Psychosocial Care
  - Use an interprofessional approach.
  - Provide care to the client and the family.
  - Provide a "turn the other way caring presence" through two essential skills: listening and observing.
  - Use volunteers when appropriate to provide nonmedical care.
  - Use therapeutic communication to develop and maintain a nurse-client relationship.
  - Facilitate understanding of information regarding disease progression and treatment choices.
  - Facilitate communication between the client, family, and provider.
  - Encourage the client to participate in religious/spiritual practices that bring comfort and strength, if appropriate.
  - Assist the client in clarifying personal values to facilitate effective decision-making.
  - Encourage the client to use coping mechanisms that have worked in the past.

  - Be sensitive to comments made in the presence of a client who is unconscious, as it is widely accepted that hearing is the last of the senses that is lost.
- Protection Against Abandonment and Isolation
  - Decrease the fear of dying alone.
    - Make presence known by answering call lights in a timely manner and making frequent contact.
    - Keep the client informed of procedure/assessment times.
    - Allow family members to spend the night.
    - Determine where the client is most comfortable, such as in a room close to the nurses' station.
- Support for the Grieving Family
  - Suggest that family members plan visits in a manner that promotes client rest.
  - Ensure that the family receives appropriate information as the treatment plan changes.
  - Provide privacy so family members have the opportunity to communicate and express feelings among themselves without including the client.
  - Determine family members' desire to provide physical care. Provide instruction as necessary.
  - Reinforce education with the family about physical changes to expect as the client moves closer to death.

POSTMORTEM CARE

Overview

- A nurse is responsible for following federal and state laws regarding requests for organ or tissue donation, obtaining permission for autopsy, certification and appropriate documentation of the death, and providing safe postmortem (after-death) care.
- The client's family now becomes the nurse's primary focus.

Nursing Interventions

- Care of the Body
  - Provide care with respect and compassion while attending to the desires of the client and family per their cultural, religious, and social practices.
  - Recognize that the provider certifies the client's death by pronouncing time and documenting therapies used, and actions taken prior to the death.
  - Preparing the body for viewing includes:
    - Maintaining privacy.
    - Shaving facial hair if applicable and/or desired by the family.
    - Removing all tubes and soiled linens, unless organs are to be donated or this is a coroner's case.
    - Removing all personal belongings to be given to the family.
    - Cleansing and positioning the body with a pillow under the head, arms outside the sheet and blanket, dentures in place, and eyes closed.
    - Applying fresh linens and a gown.
    - Brushing/combing the client's hair, replacing any hair pieces.
    - Removing excess equipment and linens from the room.
    - Dimming the lights and minimizing noise to provide a calm environment.
  - Viewing considerations include:
    - Asking the family if they would like to remain with the body, honoring any decision. This process should not be rushed.
    - Clarifying and documenting where the client's personal belongings should go either with the body or to a designated person.
    - Adhering to the same procedures when the deceased is a newborn, while adding the following.
      - Swaddling the infant's body in a clean blanket
      - Transporting the cradled infant in the nurse's arms or in a special infant carrier
      - Offering mementos of the infant (identification bracelets, footprints, cord clamp, lock of hair, photos)
  - Post viewing
    - Apply identification tags according to the facility's policy.
    - Complete documentation.
    - Remain aware of visitor and staff sensibilities during transport.
- Organ Donation
  - Recognize that request for tissue and organ donation must be made by specially trained personnel.
  - Provide support and education to family members as decisions are being made. Use a private area for any family discussions concerning donation.
  - Be sensitive to cultural and religious influences.
  - Maintain ventilatory and cardiovascular support for vital organ retrieval.

- Autopsy Considerations
  - The provider typically approaches the family about performing an autopsy.
  - The nurse's role is to answer the family's questions and support the family's choices.
  - Autopsies can be conducted to advance scientific knowledge regarding disease processes, which can lead to the development of new therapies.
  - The law can require an autopsy to be performed if the death is due to a homicide or accident, or if the death occurs within 24 hr of hospital admission.
  - Most facilities require that equipment used during medical intervention, such as tubes, remain in place if an autopsy is planned.
- Cultural/Religious Beliefs
  - Identify cultural/religious beliefs of family members.
  - Be sensitive to these practices when providing postmortem care.
- Documentation and completion of forms following federal and state laws typically includes the following.
  - Person pronouncing the death and at what time
  - Consideration of and preparation for organ donation
  - Disposition of personal articles
  - Names of people notified and any decisions made
  - Location of identification tags
  - Time the body left the facility and the destination

Care of the Nurses Who Are Grieving

- Caring long-term for a client can create personal attachments for nurses.
- Nurses can practice positive self-care by using coping strategies.
  - Attending debriefing sessions with colleagues
  - Attending the client's funeral
  - Communicating in writing to the client's family
  - Using stress-management techniques
  - Talking with a professional counselor

APPLICATION EXERCISES

1. A nurse is reviewing a newly admitted client's medical record. Which of the following documents is a directive for medical treatment based on the client's wishes?

    A. Advance directives

    B. Living will

    C. Informed consent

    D. Durable power of attorney for health care

2. A nurse is reviewing Kübler-Ross's Five Stages of Grief with a group of newly licensed nurses. Which of the following should the nurse include in the education? (Select all that apply.)

_____ A. Endurance

_____ B. Denial

_____ C. Bargaining

_____ D. Anger

_____ E. Depression

3. A nurse is working with a client who has recently lost his mother. The nurse recognizes that which of the following factors influence grief and coping ability? (Select all that apply.)

_____ A. Interpersonal relationships

_____ B. Culture

_____ C. Birth order

_____ D. Size of family

_____ E. Prior experience with loss

4. A nurse is discussing normal uncomplicated grief with a client who recently lost a child. Which of the following statements made by the client requires additional intervention?

    A. "I may experience feelings of resentment."

    B. "I may withdraw from others."

    C. "It is possible to experience changes in sleep."

    D. "It is possible to experience suicidal thoughts."

5. A nurse is caring for a client who lost his mother to cancer last month. Which of the following statements made by the nurse is a nontherapeutic response?

    A. "You sound angry. Anger is a normal feeling associated with loss."

    B. "Tell me more about how you are feeling."

    C. "I understand just how you feel. I felt the same when my mother died."

    D. "Let's discuss how you have been coping."

6. A nurse is caring for a client who is dying. Use the ATI Active Learning Template: Basic Concept to complete this item by identifying at least three nursing interventions that the nurse can use to assist the client to maintain dignity and self-esteem during end-of-life care.

APPLICATION EXERCISES KEY

1.   A. INCORRECT: Advance directives are legal documents that direct end-of-life issues.

     B. **CORRECT:** Living wills are documents that direct medical treatment based on the client's wishes.

     C. INCORRECT: Informed consent is a process of getting permission from a client to perform test or procedures.

     D. INCORRECT: Durable power of attorney for health care is a document that appoints an individual to make medical decisions when a client is no longer able to do so on his own behalf.

     (N) NCLEX® Connection: Coordinated Care, Legal Responsibilities

2.   A. INCORRECT: Endurance is a component of the Styles of Confronting the Prospect of Dying: Seven Motifs. Individuals are determined to continue on with life and take control as they are dying.

     B. **CORRECT:** Denial is having difficulty believing a terminal diagnosis or loss. This is one of Kübler-Ross Five Stages of Grief.

     C. **CORRECT:** Bargaining is when the client negotiates for more time or a cure. This is one of Kübler-Ross Five Stages of Grief.

     D. **CORRECT:** Anger is directed toward self, others, or objects. This is one of Kübler-Ross Five Stages of Grief.

     E. **CORRECT:** Depression is when the client is saddened over the inability to change the situation.

     (N) NCLEX® Connection: Psychosocial Integrity, End of Life Concepts

3.   A. **CORRECT:** Interpersonal relationships are factors that influence grief and ability to cope.

     B. **CORRECT:** Culture is a factor that influences grief and ability to cope.

     C. INCORRECT: Birth order is not a factor that influences grief and ability to cope.

     D. INCORRECT: Family size is not a factor that influences grief and ability to cope.

     E. **CORRECT:** Prior experience with loss is a factor that influences grief and ability to cope.

     (N) NCLEX® Connection: Psychosocial Integrity, End of Life Concepts

4. A. INCORRECT: Resentment is an emotion that can be associated with normal uncomplicated grief. Therefore, this does not require further intervention by the nurse.

   B. INCORRECT: Withdrawal is an emotion that can be seen with normal uncomplicated grief. Therefore, this does not require further intervention by the nurse.

   C. INCORRECT: Somatic complaints such as changes in sleep patterns can be associated with normal uncomplicated grief. Therefore, this does not require further intervention by the nurse.

   D. **CORRECT:** Suicidal ideations are associated with dysfunctional grieving. Therefore, this response requires additional nursing intervention.

   Ⓝ NCLEX® Connection: Psychosocial Integrity, End of Life Concepts

5. A. INCORRECT: This is a therapeutic response that acknowledges the client's emotion.

   B. INCORRECT: This is an open-ended therapeutic response that allows the client to take the direction of the discussion.

   C. **CORRECT:** This is a closed-ended nontherapeutic statement. This is an example of minimizing feelings. The nurse implies that she knows just how the client feels, which is not always true.

   D. INCORRECT: This is a therapeutic response that offers general leads for the communication.

   Ⓝ NCLEX® Connection: Psychosocial Integrity, Therapeutic Communication

6. *Using the ATI Active Learning Template: Basic Concept*
   - Nursing Interventions
     - Listen to the client's concerns.
     - Maintain cleanliness and odor control in the client's physical environment.
     - Allow the client to participate in ADLs as desired.
     - Provide personal grooming assistance as necessary.
     - Encourage the client to make decisions regarding food selection, activities, and health care.

   Ⓝ NCLEX® Connection: Psychosocial Integrity, End of Life Concepts

chapter 26

Overview

- Mental health and developmental disorders in children and adolescents are not always easily diagnosed, resulting in possible delayed or inadequate treatment interventions. Factors that contribute to this include the following.
  - Children might not have the ability or the necessary skills to describe what is happening.
  - Children demonstrate a wide variation of "normal" behaviors, especially in different developmental stages.
  - It is difficult to determine whether a child's behavior indicates an emotional problem.
- A child's behavior is problematic when it interferes with home, school, and interactions with peers.
  - Behaviors are considered pathologic when they
    - Are not age-appropriate.
    - Deviate from cultural norms.
    - Create deficits or impairments in adaptive functioning.
- Disorders that can appear during childhood and adolescence include the following.
  - Depressive disorders, such as major depressive disorder and dysthymic disorder
  - Anxiety disorders, including separation anxiety disorder and panic disorder
  - Trauma- and stressor-related disorders, such as posttraumatic stress disorder (PTSD)
  - Substance use disorders, such as alcohol use disorder, tobacco use disorder, and cannabis use disorder
  - Feeding and eating disorders, such as anorexia nervosa, bulimia nervosa, and binge eating disorder
  - Disruptive, impulse control, and conduct disorders, such as oppositional defiant disorder, disruptive mood dysregulation disorder, and conduct disorder
  - Neurodevelopmental disorders, including attention deficit/hyperactivity disorder (ADHD), autism spectrum disorder, intellectual developmental disorder, and specific learning disorder
  - Bipolar and related disorders
  - Schizophrenia spectrum and other psychotic disorders
  - Nonsuicidal self-injury and suicidal behavior disorder (suicide is a leading cause of death for youth between the ages of 10 and 24)

- Childhood and adolescent disorders can have associated comorbid conditions and can meet the criteria for more than one mental health disorder.
- The characteristics of good mental health for a child and adolescent include the following.
  - Ability to appropriately interpret reality, as well as having a correct perception of the surrounding environment
  - Positive self-concept
  - Ability to cope with stress and anxiety in an age-appropriate way
  - Mastery of developmental tasks
  - Ability to express oneself spontaneously and creatively
  - Ability to develop and maintain satisfying relationships

Data Collection

- Etiology and General Risk Factors
  - Genetic links or chromosomal abnormalities are associated with some disorders such as schizophrenia, bipolar disorder, autism spectrum disorder, ADHD, and intellectual developmental disorder.
  - Biochemical – Alterations in neurotransmitters, including norepinephrine, serotonin, or dopamine, contribute to some mental health disorders.
  - Social and environmental – Severe marital discord, low socioeconomic status, large families and overcrowding, parental criminality, substance use disorders, maternal psychiatric disorders, parental depression, and foster care placement are all risk factors.
  - Cultural and ethnic – Difficulty with assimilation, lack of cultural role models, and lack of support from the dominant culture can contribute to mental health issues.
  - Resiliency – The ability to adapt to changes in the environment, form nurturing relationships, distance oneself from the emotional chaos of the parent or family, model effective coping strategies, and use problem-solving skills can help an at-risk child avoid the development of a mental health disorder.
  - Witnessing or experiencing traumatic events, such as physical or sexual abuse, during the formative years are risk factors.

Depressive Disorders

- Risk factors associated with childhood or adolescent depression include the following.
  - Family history of depression
  - Physical or sexual abuse or neglect
  - Homelessness
  - Disputes among parents, conflicts with peers or family, and rejection by peers or family
  - Bullying, either as the aggressor or victim, including both traditional bullying and cyberbullying behavior

- ○ Engaging in high-risk behaviors
- ○ Learning disabilities
- ○ Having a chronic illness
- Subjective and Objective Data
  - ○ Feelings of sadness
  - ○ Loss of appetite
  - ○ Nonspecific complaints related to health
  - ○ Engaging in solitary play or work
  - ○ Changes in appetite resulting in weight changes
  - ○ Changes in sleeping patterns
  - ○ Irritability
  - ○ Aggression
  - ○ High-risk behavior
  - ○ Poor school performance and/or dropping out of school
  - ○ Feelings of hopelessness about the future
  - ○ Suicidal ideation or suicide attempts

Anxiety Disorders and Trauma- and Stressor-Related Disorders

- Subjective and Objective Data
  - ○ The anxiety or level of stress interferes with normal growth and development.
  - ○ The anxiety or level of stress is so serious that the child is unable to function normally at home, in school, and in other areas of life.
- Separation Anxiety Disorder
  - ○ This type of disorder is characterized by excessive anxiety when a child is separated from or anticipating separation from home or parents. The anxiety can develop into a school phobia or phobia of being left alone. Depression is also common.
  - ○ Anxiety can develop after a specific stressor (death of a relative or pet, an illness, a move, an assault).
  - ○ Anxiety can progress to a panic disorder or type of phobia.
- Posttraumatic Stress Disorder (PTSD)
  - ○ PTSD is precipitated by experiencing, witnessing, or learning of a traumatic event.
  - ○ Children and adolescents who have PTSD exhibit psychologic indications of anxiety, depression, phobia, or conversion reactions.
  - ○ If the anxiety resulting from PTSD is displayed externally, it is often manifested as irritability and aggression with family and friends, poor academic performance, somatic reports, belief that life will be short, and difficulty sleeping.

Disruptive, Impulse Control, and Conduct Disorders

- Subjective and Objective Data
  - Behavioral problems usually occur in school, church, home, and/or recreational activities.
  - In children and adolescents who have disruptive, impulse control, and conduct disorders, clinical manifestations generally worsen in the following.
    - Situations that require sustained attention, such as in the classroom
    - Unstructured group situations, such as the playground
- Oppositional Defiant Disorder
  - This disorder is characterized by a recurrent pattern of the following antisocial behaviors.
    - Negativity
    - Disobedience
    - Hostility
    - Defiant behaviors (especially toward authority figures)
    - Stubbornness
    - Argumentativeness
    - Limit testing
    - Unwillingness to compromise
    - Refusal to accept responsibility for misbehavior
  - Misbehavior usually is demonstrated at home and directed toward the person best known.
  - Children and adolescents who have oppositional defiant disorder do not see themselves as defiant. They view their behavior as a response to unreasonable demands and/or circumstances.
  - Clients who have this disorder can exhibit low self-esteem, mood lability, and a low frustration threshold.
  - Oppositional defiant disorder can develop into conduct disorder.
- Disruptive Mood Dysregulation Disorder
  - Clients who have this disorder exhibit recurrent temper outbursts that are severe and do not correlate with situation.
    - Temper outbursts are manifested verbally and/or physically and can include aggression.
    - Temper outbursts are not appropriate for the client's developmental level.
  - Temper outbursts are present three or more times per week and are observable by others, such as parents, peers, and teachers, in at least two settings, such as home and school.
  - Onset of this disorder is between the ages of 6 and 10.
  - Clinical manifestations are not due to another mental health disorder such as bipolar disorder.

- Conduct Disorder (Childhood or Adolescent-Onset Type)
  - Clients who have conduct disorder demonstrate a persistent pattern of behavior that violates the rights of others or rules and norms of society. Categories of conduct disorder include the following.
    - Aggression to people and animals
    - Destruction of property
    - Deceitfulness or theft
    - Serious violations of rules

CONDUCT DISORDER	
Contributing Factors	Manifestations
› Parental rejection and neglect	› Demonstrates a lack of remorse or care for the feelings of others
› Difficult infant temperament	› Bullies, threatens, and intimidates others
› Inconsistent child-rearing practices with harsh discipline	› Believes that aggression is justified
› Physical or sexual abuse	› Exhibits low self-esteem, irritability, temper outbursts, reckless behavior
› Lack of supervision	› Can demonstrate signs of suicidal ideation
› Early institutionalization	› Can have concurrent learning disorders or impairments in cognitive functioning
› Frequent changing of caregivers	› Demonstrates physical cruelty to others and/or animals
› Large family size	› Has used a weapon that could cause serious injuries
› Association with delinquent peer groups	› Destroys property of others
› Parent with a history of psychological illness	› Has run away from home
	› Often lies, shoplifts, and is truant from school

Neurodevelopmental Disorders

- Attention deficit hyperactivity disorder (ADHD) involves the inability of a person to control behaviors requiring sustained attention.
  - Inattention, impulsivity, and hyperactivity are characteristic behaviors of ADHD.
    - Inattention is evidenced by a difficulty in paying attention, listening, and focusing.
    - Hyperactivity is evidenced by fidgeting, an inability to sit still, running and climbing inappropriately, difficulty with playing quietly, and talking excessively.
    - Impulsivity is evidenced by difficulty waiting for turns, constantly interrupting others, and acting without the consideration of consequences.
  - Inattentive or impulsive behavior can put the child at risk for injury.
  - Behaviors associated with ADHD must be present prior to age 12 and must be present in more than one setting to be diagnosed as ADHD. Behaviors associated with ADHD can receive negative attention from adults and peers.
  - Types of ADHD include the following.
    - Combined type – Client exhibits both inattentive and hyperactive-impulsive behaviors.
    - ADHD predominantly inattentive.
    - ADHD predominantly hyperactive-impulsive.

- Autism Spectrum Disorder
    - Autism spectrum disorder is a complex neurodevelopmental disorder thought to be of genetic origin with a wide spectrum of behaviors affecting an individual's ability to communicate and interact with others. Cognitive and language development typically are delayed. Characteristic behaviors include inability to maintain eye contact, repetitive actions, and strict observance of routines.
    - This type of disorder is present in early childhood and is more common in boys than girls.
    - Physical difficulties experienced by the child who has autism spectrum disorder include sensory integration dysfunction, sleep disorders, digestive disorders, feeding disorders, epilepsy, and/or allergies.
    - There is a wide variability in functioning. Abilities can range from poor (inability to perform self-care, inability to communicate and relate to others) to high (ability to function at near-normal levels).
- Intellectual Developmental Disorder
    - Clients who have intellectual developmental disorder have an onset of deficits and impairments during the developmental period of infancy or childhood.
    - The client has intellectual deficits with mental abilities such as reasoning, abstract thinking, academic learning, and learning from prior experiences.
    - Clients demonstrate impaired ability to maintain personal independence and social responsibility, including activities of daily living, social participation, and the need for ongoing support at school.
- Specific Learning Disorder
    - Client demonstrates persistent difficulty in acquiring reading, writing, or mathematical skills.
    - Performance in one or more of the academic areas is significantly lower than the average range for the client's age, level of intelligence, or educational level.
    - Clients who have specific learning disorder benefit from an individualized education program (IEP).

Patient-Centered Care

- Nursing Care
    - Obtain a complete nursing history.
        - Mother's pregnancy and birth history
        - Sleeping, eating, and elimination patterns; recent weight loss or gain
        - Achievement of developmental milestones
        - Allergies
        - Current medications
        - Peer and family relationships, school performance
        - History of emotional, physical, or sexual abuse
        - Parental perceptions and level of tolerance toward child's behavior
        - Family history, including current members of the household
        - Substance use
            - Tobacco use disorder, such as cigarettes, cigars, snuff, chewing tobacco
            - Alcohol, frequency of use, driving under the influence, and family history of alcohol use disorder
            - Drugs (illegal or prescription) to get high, stay calm, lose weight, or stay awake

- Safety at home and at school
- Actual or potential risk for self-injury
- Presence of depression and suicidal ideation, including a plan, the lethality of that plan, and the means to carry out the plan
- Availability of weapons in the home

○ Assist with performing data collection, including a mental status examination.

○ Use primary prevention, such as education, peer group discussions, and mentoring to prevent risky behavior and to promote healthy behavior and effective coping.

- Work with clients to adopt a realistic view of their bodies and to improve overall self-esteem.
- Identify and reinforce the use of positive coping skills.
- Employ the use of gun and weapon control strategies.
- Emphasize the use of seat belts when in motor vehicles.
- Encourage the use of protective gear for high-impact sports.
- Discuss contraceptives and other sexual information, such as the transmission and prevention of HIV and other sexually transmitted infections.
- Encourage abstinence, but keep the lines of communication open to allow the adolescent to discuss sexual practices.
- Encourage clients and family members to seek professional help if indicated.

○ Intervene for clients who have engaged in high-risk behaviors.

- Reinforce teaching to the client and family on factors that contribute to substance use disorders. Make appropriate referrals when indicated.
- Inform the client and family about support groups in the community for eating disorders, substance use disorders, and general teen support.
- Reinforce teaching with the client regarding individuals within the school environment and community to whom concerns can be voiced about personal safety and bullying, such as police officers, school nurses, counselors, and teachers.
- Discuss referral to social services with the charge nurse when indicated.
- Discuss the use and availability of support hotlines.

- Perform a depression and suicide assessment. Make an immediate referral for professional care when indicated.

- Interventions for Anxiety Disorders

  ○ Providing emotional support that is accepting of regression and other defense mechanisms

  ○ Offering protection during panic levels of anxiety by providing for needs

  ○ Implementing methods to increase client self-esteem and feelings of achievement

- Interventions for Trauma- and Stressor-Related Disorders

  ○ Providing assistance with working through traumatic events or losses to reach acceptance

  ○ Encouraging group therapy

- Interventions for Disruptive, Impulse Control, and Conduct Disorders, and ADHD
  - Use a calm, firm, respectful approach with the child.
  - Use modeling to show acceptable behavior.
  - Obtain the child's attention before giving directions. Provide short and clear explanations.
  - Set clear limits on unacceptable behaviors and be consistent.
  - Plan physical activities through which the child can use energy and obtain success.
  - Assist parents to develop a reward system using methods such as a wall chart or tokens. Encourage the child to participate.
  - Focus on the family and child's strengths, not just the problems.
  - Support the parents' efforts to remain hopeful.
  - Provide a safe environment for the child and others.
  - Provide the child with specific positive feedback when expectations are met.
  - Identify issues that result in power struggles.
  - Assist the child in developing effective coping mechanisms.
  - Encourage the child to participate in group, individual, and family therapy.
  - Administer medications, such as antipsychotics, mood stabilizers, anticonvulsants, and antidepressants. Monitor for side effects.
- Interventions for Autism Spectrum Disorder
  - Discuss referral for early intervention.
  - Provide for a structured environment.
  - Consult with parents to provide consistent and individualized care.
  - Encourage parents to participate in the child's care and treatment plan as much as possible.
  - Use short, concise, and developmentally appropriate communication.
  - Identify desired behaviors and reward them.
  - Role-model social skills.
  - Role-play situations that involve conflict and conflict-resolution strategies.
  - Encourage verbal communication.
  - Limit self-stimulating and ritualistic behaviors by providing alternative play activities.
  - Determine emotional and situational triggers.
  - Give plenty of notice before changing routines.
  - Carefully monitor the child's behaviors to ensure safety.

- Teamwork and Collaboration

  ○ Family therapy enables the client and entire family to address problems.

  ○ Cognitive-behavioral therapy (CBT) is useful to change negative thoughts to positive outcomes when intervening for depressive, disruptive, impulse control, and conduct disorders.

  ○ Grief and trauma intervention (GTI) for children is effective for clients who have a trauma- and stressor-related disorder. GTI encourages narrative expression, such as drawing, writing, or play regarding the traumatic event.

  ○ Other therapeutic approaches can include group therapy, play therapy, mutual storytelling, therapeutic games, bibliotherapy, and therapeutic drawing.

- Medications

  ○ Medications for children and adolescents include CNS stimulants, such as methylphenidate (Concerta, Ritalin SR); norepinephrine selective reuptake inhibitors, such as atomoxetine (Strattera); tricyclic antidepressants, such as desipramine (Norpramin); alpha$_2$-adrenergic agonists, such as guanfacine (Intuniv); and antipsychotics-atypical, such as risperidone (Risperdal).

APPLICATION EXERCISES

1. A nurse is assisting the parents of a school-age child who has oppositional defiant disorder in identifying strategies to promote positive behavior. Which of the following are appropriate strategies for the nurse to recommend? (Select all that apply.)

      _____ A. Allow the child to choose consequences for negative behavior.

      _____ B. Use role-playing to act out unacceptable behavior.

      _____ C. Develop a reward system for acceptable behavior.

      _____ D. Encourage the child to participate in school sports.

      _____ E. Be consistent when addressing unacceptable behavior.

2. A nurse is collecting data on an adolescent client who has depression. Which of the following are expected findings? (Select all that apply.)

      _____ A. Fear of being alone

      _____ B. Substance use

      _____ C. Weight gain

      _____ D. Irritability

      _____ E. Aggressiveness

3. A nurse working in a pediatric clinic is caring for a preschool-age child who has a new diagnosis of ADHD. When reinforcing teaching with the parent about this disorder, which of the following statements should the nurse include in the teaching?

A. "Behaviors associated with ADHD must be present prior to age 3."

B. "This disorder is characterized by argumentativeness."

C. "Below-average intellectual functioning is associated with ADHD."

D. "Because of this disorder, your child is at an increased risk for injury."

4. A nurse is assisting with obtaining a health history from the parents of a 12-year-old client who has conduct disorder. Which of the following are expected findings? (Select all that apply.)

_____ A. Bullying of others

_____ B. Threats of suicide

_____ C. Law-breaking activities

_____ D. Narcissistic behavior

_____ E. Flat affect

5. A nurse is collecting data on a 4-year-old child for indications of autism spectrum disorder. For which of the following indications should the nurse monitor?

A. Impulsive behavior

B. Repetitive counting

C. Destructiveness

D. Somatic problems

6. A nurse is assisting with conducting a peer group discussion with a group of high school students about primary prevention. Use the ATI Active Learning Template: Basic Concept to complete this item to include the following sections:

A. Underlying Principles: Identify the underlying purpose of primary prevention.

B. Nursing Interventions: Identify at least four primary prevention interventions.

APPLICATION EXERCISES KEY

1. A. INCORRECT: The parents should set clear limits on unacceptable behavior.

    B. INCORRECT: The parents should focus on acceptable behavior and demonstrate this through modeling.

    C. **CORRECT:** The parents should have a method to reward the child for acceptable behavior.

    D. **CORRECT:** The parents should encourage physical activity through which the child can use energy and obtain success.

    E. **CORRECT:** The parents should set clear limits on unacceptable behavior and be consistent.

    (N) NCLEX® Connection: Psychosocial Integrity, Behavioral Management

2. A. INCORRECT: Solitary play or work, rather than the fear of being alone, is an expected finding associated with depression.

    B. **CORRECT:** Substance use is an expected finding associated with depression.

    C. INCORRECT: Loss of appetite and weight loss, not weight gain, are expected findings associated with depression.

    D. **CORRECT:** Irritability is an expected finding associated with depression.

    E. **CORRECT:** Aggressiveness is an expected finding associated with depression.

    (N) NCLEX® Connection: Psychosocial Integrity, Mental Health Concepts

3. A. INCORRECT: Behaviors associated with ADHD must be present before the age of 12.

    B. INCORRECT: Argumentativeness is associated with oppositional defiant disorder rather than ADHD.

    C. INCORRECT: Below-average intellectual functioning is associated with intellectual developmental disorder rather than ADHD.

    D. **CORRECT:** Inattentive or impulsive behavior increases the risk for injury in a child who has ADHD.

    (N) NCLEX® Connection: Psychosocial Integrity, Behavioral Management

4. A. **CORRECT:** Bullying behavior is an expected finding of conduct disorder.

   B. **CORRECT:** Suicidal ideation is an expected finding of conduct disorder.

   C. **CORRECT:** Law- and/or rule-breaking behavior is an expected finding of conduct disorder.

   D. INCORRECT: Low self-esteem, rather than narcissism, is an expected finding of conduct disorder.

   E. INCORRECT: Irritability and temper outbursts, rather than a flat affect, are expected findings of conduct disorder.

   Ⓝ NCLEX® Connection: Psychosocial Integrity, Mental Health Concepts

5. A. INCORRECT: Impulsive behavior is an indication of ADHD rather than autism spectrum disorder.

   B. **CORRECT:** Repetitive actions and strict routines are an indication of autism spectrum disorder.

   C. INCORRECT: Destructiveness is an indication of conduct disorder rather than autism spectrum disorder.

   D. INCORRECT: Somatic problems are an indication of posttraumatic stress disorder rather than autism spectrum disorder.

   Ⓝ NCLEX® Connection: Psychosocial Integrity, Mental Health Concepts

6. *Using ATI Active Learning Template: Basic Concept*

   A. Underlying Principles
   - The purpose of primary prevention is to help the adolescent avoid risky behavior and to promote healthy behavior and effective coping.

   B. Nursing Interventions
   - Assist clients in adopting a realistic view of their bodies.
   - Promote positive self-esteem.
   - Identify and reinforce the use of positive coping skills.
   - Employ the use of gun- and weapon-control strategies.
   - Emphasize the use of seat belts when in motor vehicles.
   - Encourage the use of protective gear for high-impact sports.
   - Reinforce teaching regarding use of contraceptives and the prevention of sexually transmitted infections.

   Ⓝ NCLEX® Connection: Health Promotion and Maintenance, High Risk Behaviors

Psychiatric Emergencies

CHAPTERS

› Crisis Management
› Suicide
› Anger Management
› Family and Community Violence

NCLEX® CONNECTIONS

When reviewing the chapters in this unit, keep in mind the relevant sections of the NCLEX® outline, in particular:

Client Needs: Psychosocial Integrity

› Relevant topics/tasks include:

» Crisis Intervention

› Identify a client in crisis.

› Use crisis intervention techniques to assist the client in coping.

› Identify the client's risk for self injury and/or violence (suicide or violence precautions).

» Abuse or Neglect

› Recognize risk factors for domestic, child and/or elder abuse/neglect, and sexual abuse.

› Reinforce client teaching on coping strategies to prevent abuse or neglect.

chapter 27

Overview

- A crisis is an acute, time-limited (usually lasting 4 to 6 weeks) event during which a client experiences an emotional response that cannot be managed with the client's normal coping mechanisms.
- Everyone experiences crises. A crisis is not pathological, but represents a struggle for equilibrium and adaptation.
- Crises are also personal in nature. What is considered a crisis for one person might not be so for another.
- Common characteristics include:
  - Experience of a sudden event with little or no time to prepare.
  - Perception of the event as overwhelming or life-threatening.
  - Loss or decrease in communication with significant others.
  - Sense of displacement from the familiar.
  - An actual or perceived loss.
- Types of crises include:
  - Situational/external – often unanticipated loss or change experienced in everyday, often unanticipated, life events.
  - Maturational/internal – achieving new developmental stages, which requires learning additional coping mechanisms.
  - Adventitious – the occurrence of natural disasters, crimes, or national disasters.
    - People in communities with large-scale psychological trauma caused by natural disasters

Data Collection

- Risk and Protective Factors
  - Accumulation of unresolved losses
  - Current life stressors
  - Concurrent mental and physical health issues
  - Excessive fatigue or pain
  - Age and developmental stage
  - Support system
  - Prior experience with stress/crisis

- Subjective/Objective Data
  - The nursing history should include the following.
    - Presence of suicidal or homicidal ideation requiring hospitalization
    - The client's perception of the precipitating event
    - Cultural or religious needs of the client
    - Support system
    - Present coping skills
  - Phases of a crisis

PHASE	MANIFESTATIONS
Phase 1	› Escalating anxiety from a threat activates increased defense responses.
Phase 2	› Anxiety continues escalating as defense responses fail, functioning becomes disorganized, and the client resorts to trial-and-error attempts to resolve anxiety.
Phase 3	› Trial-and-error methods of resolution fail and the client's anxiety escalates to severe or panic levels, leading to flight or withdrawal behaviors.
Phase 4	› The client experiences overwhelming anxiety that can lead to anguish and apprehension, feelings of powerlessness and being overwhelmed, dissociative symptoms (depersonalization, detachment from reality), depression, confusion, and/or violence against others or self.

Patient-Centered Care

- Nursing Care
  - Crisis intervention is designed to provide rapid assistance for individuals or groups who have an urgent need.
  - Initial task of nurse is to promote a sense of safety by determining the client's potential for suicide or homicide.
  - Initial nursing interventions include:
    - Identifying the current problem and directing interventions for resolution.
    - Taking an active, directive role with the client.
    - Helping the client to set realistic, attainable goals.
  - Critical Incident Stress Debriefing (CISD) is a group approach that can be used with a group of people who have been exposed to a crisis situation.

- ○ Provide for client safety.
  - ▪ Initiate hospitalization to protect clients who have suicidal or homicidal thoughts.
  - ▪ Prioritize interventions to address the client's physical needs first.
- ○ Use strategies to decrease anxiety.
  - ▪ Develop a therapeutic nurse-client relationship.
    - □ Remain with the client.
    - □ Listen and observe.
    - □ Make eye contact.
    - □ Ask questions related to the client's feelings.
    - □ Ask questions related to the event.
    - □ Demonstrate genuineness and caring.
    - □ Communicate clearly and, if needed, with clear directives.
    - □ Avoid false reassurance and other nontherapeutic responses.
- ○ Encourage relaxation techniques.
- ○ Identify and discuss coping skills (assertiveness training and parenting skills).
- ○ Assist the client with the development of the following type of action plan.
  - ▪ Short-term, no longer than 24 to 72 hr
  - ▪ Focused on the crisis
  - ▪ Realistic and manageable
- • Medications
  - ○ Administer antianxiety and/or antidepressant medication as prescribed.
- • Client Education

  - ○ Identify and coordinate with support agencies and other resources.
  - ○ Plan and provide for follow-up care.

APPLICATION EXERCISES

1. A nurse is conducting chart reviews of multiple clients at a community mental health facility. Which of the following would be an example of client experiencing a maturational crisis?

    A. Rape

    B. Marriage

    C. Severe physical illness

    D. Job loss

2. A nurse is caring for a client who is experiencing a crisis. Which of the following medications might the provider prescribe? (Select all that apply.)

_____ A. Lithium carbonate (Lithobid)

_____ B. Paroxetine (Paxil)

_____ C. Risperidone (Risperdal)

_____ D. Haloperidol (Haldol)

_____ E. Lorazepam (Ativan)

3. A nurse is assisting with an in-service on crisis management for a group of newly licensed emergency care nurses. Use the ATI Active Learning Template: Basic Concept to complete this item by identifying three nursing interventions that the nurse can use to assist the client who is experiencing a crisis.

APPLICATION EXERCISES KEY

1.   A. INCORRECT: Rape is an example of an adventitious crisis. It is not a part of everyday life.

   B. **CORRECT:** Marriage is a example of a maturational crisis, which is naturally occurring across the life span.

   C. INCORRECT: Severe physical illness is an example of a situational crisis.

   D. INCORRECT: Loss of a job is an example of a situational crisis.

   Ⓝ NCLEX® Connection: Psychosocial Integrity, Crisis Intervention

2.   A. INCORRECT: Lithobid is a mood stabilizer prescribed for bipolar disorder.

   B. **CORRECT:** Paxil is an antidepressant and can be prescribed for the depression that can follow a crisis situation.

   C. INCORRECT: Antipsychotic medications can be prescribed for disturbed thought processes, usually when accompanied by other psychotic symptoms (hallucinations, delusions, blunt affect). Antipsychotics are not indicated in a short-term crisis situation.

   D. INCORRECT: Antipsychotic medications can be prescribed for disturbed thought processes, usually when accompanied by other psychotic symptoms (hallucinations, delusions, blunt affect). Antipsychotics are not indicated in a short-term crisis situation.

   E. **CORRECT:** A benzodiazepine can be useful to minimize the anxiety that a client might feel in a crisis situation.

   Ⓝ NCLEX® Connection: Pharmacological Therapies, Expected Actions/Outcomes

3.   *Using the ATI Active Learning Template: Basic Concept*
   • Nursing Interventions
     ○ Identify the current problem and direct interventions for resolution.
     ○ Take an active, directive role with the client.
     ○ Help the client to set realistic, attainable goals.
     ○ Provide for client safety.
     ○ Initiate hospitalization to protect clients who have suicidal or homicidal thoughts.
     ○ Prioritize interventions to address the client's physical needs first.
     ○ Use strategies to decrease anxiety.
     ○ Develop a therapeutic nurse-client relationship.
     ○ Provide instructions on relaxation techniques.
     ○ Encourage coping skills.
     ○ Administer prescribed antianxiety and/or antidepressant medications.

   Ⓝ NCLEX® Connection: Psychosocial Integrity, Crisis Intervention

chapter 28

Overview

- Suicide is the intentional act of killing oneself.

- A client who is suicidal may be ambivalent about death. Intervention can make a difference.

- A client contemplating suicide believes that the act is the end to problems. Little concern is given to the aftermath and the ramifications to those left behind. Long-term therapy is needed for the survivors.

- Suicidal ideation occurs when a client is having thoughts about committing suicide.

- Myths regarding suicide

  ○ People who talk about suicide never commit it.

  ○ People who are suicidal only want to hurt themselves, not others.

  ○ There is no way to help someone who really wants to kill himself.

  ○ Mention of the word suicide will cause the suicidal individual to actually commit suicide.

  ○ Ignoring verbal threats of suicide, or challenging a person to carry out suicide plans, will reduce the individual's use of these behaviors.

  ○ People who talk about suicide are only trying to get attention.

- Levels of Nursing Intervention

  ○ Primary – prevention strategies that include providing information and education to at-risk populations

  ○ Secondary – management of the suicide crisis

  ○ Tertiary – interventions with the family or friends of a person who committed suicide

Data Collection

- Risk Factors

  ○ Those at highest risk for suicide include adolescent, young adult, and older adult males; and persons who have comorbid mental illness, such as depressive disorders, anxiety disorders, substance use disorder, schizophrenia, eating disorders, bipolar disorder, and personality disorders.

  ○ Untreated depression increases the risk of suicide in the older adult client. Other risk factors for the older adult client include loss of employment and finances, feelings of isolation, powerlessness, prior attempts at suicide (older adult clients are more likely to succeed), change in functional ability, alcohol or other substance dependency, and loss of loved ones.

- ○ Biological factors
  - ▪ Family history of suicide
  - ▪ Physical disorders, such as AIDS, cancer, cardiovascular disease, stroke, chronic kidney failure, cirrhosis, dementia, epilepsy, head injury, Huntington's disease, and multiple sclerosis
- ○ Psychosocial factors
  - ▪ Sense of hopelessness
  - ▪ Intense emotions, such as rage, anger, or guilt
  - ▪ Poor interpersonal relationships at home, school, and work
  - ▪ Developmental stressors, such as those experienced by adolescents
- • Protective Factors
  - ○ Feelings of responsibility toward family
  - ○ Current pregnancy
  - ○ Religious and cultural beliefs
  - ○ Overall satisfaction with life
  - ○ Presence of adequate social support
  - ○ Effective coping and problem-solving skills
  - ○ Access to appropriate medical care
- • Subjective Data
  - ○ Check carefully for verbal and nonverbal clues. It is essential to ask the client if he is thinking of suicide. This will not give the client the idea to commit suicide.
  - ○ Suicidal comments usually are made to someone that the client perceives as supportive.
  - ○ Comments or signals can be overt or covert.
    - ▪ Overt comment – "There is just no reason for me to go on living."
    - ▪ Covert comment – "Everything is looking pretty grim for me."
  - ○ Review the client's suicide plan.
    - ▪ Does the client have a plan?
    - ▪ How lethal is the plan?
    - ▪ Can the client describe the plan exactly?
    - ▪ Does the client have access to the intended method?
    - ▪ Has the client's mood changed? A sudden change in mood from sad and depressed to happy and peaceful can indicate a client's intention to commit suicide.
- • Objective Data
  - ○ Lacerations, scratches, and scars that could indicate previous attempts at self-harm
- • Standardized Assessment Tool
  - ○ The SAD PERSONS scale is a simple and practical tool that assesses 10 major risk factors for suicide and assigns scores for each.
  - ○ It allows the triaging of suicidal clients to determine the necessity of hospitalization. Another important area to consider, not included in this tool, is the individual's intake of illicit or prescribed drugs.

Patient-Centered Care

- Nursing Care
  - Self-assessment
    - The nurse must determine how she feels personally about suicide.
    - The nurse must become comfortable asking personal questions about suicidal ideation and following up on a client's answers.
    - Death of a client by suicide can cause health care professionals to experience a hopelessness, helplessness, ambivalence, anger, anxiety, avoidance, and denial.
    - Nurses who work with suicidal clients can benefit personally by debriefing, sharing, and collaborating with other health professionals.
  - Suicide precautions include milieu therapy within the facility.
    - Initiate one-on-one constant supervision around the clock, always having the client in sight and close.
    - Document the client's location, mood, quoted statements, and behavior every 15 min or per facility protocol.
    - Remove all glass, metal silverware, electrical cords, vases, belts, shoelaces, metal nail files, tweezers, matches, razors, perfume, shampoo, and plastic bags from the client's room and vicinity.
    - Allow the client to use only plastic eating utensils.
    - Check the environment for possible hazards (such as windows that open, overhead pipes that are easily accessible.)
    - During observation periods, always check the client's hands, especially if they are hidden from sight.
    - Do not assign to a private room if possible. Keep door open at all times.
    - Ensure that the client swallows all medications.
    - Identify whether the client's current medications can be lethal with overdose. If so, collaborate with the provider to have less dangerous medications substituted if possible.
    - Restrict the visitors from bringing possibly harmful items to the client.
  - Therapeutic communication
    - When questioning the client about suicide, always use a follow-up question if the first answer is negative. For example: the client says, "I'm feeling completely hopeless." The nurse says, "Are you thinking of suicide?" Client: "No, I'm just sad." Nurse: "I can see you're very sad. Are you thinking about hurting yourself?" Client: "Well, I've thought about it a lot."
    - Establish a trusting therapeutic relationship.
    - Limit the amount of time an at-risk client spends alone.
    - Involve significant others in the treatment plan.
    - Carry out treatment plans for the client who has comorbid disorders, such as a dual diagnosis of substance use disorder.

○ Medications to prevent suicide

CLASSIFICATIONS OF MEDICATIONS TO PREVENT SUICIDE

MEDICATION EXAMPLE	CLIENT TEACHING
Antidepressants: Selective Serotonin Reuptake Inhibitors (SSRIs)	
› Citalopram (Celexa) › Fluoxetine (Prozac) › Sertraline (Zoloft)	› Do not stop taking medication suddenly. › Medications can take 1 to 3 weeks for therapeutic effects for initial response, with up to 2 months for maximal response. › Avoid hazardous activities (driving, operating heavy equipment/machinery) until medication side effects are known. Side effects can include nausea, headache, and CNS stimulation (agitation, insomnia, anxiety). › Sexual dysfunction can occur. Notify the provider if effects are intolerable. › Follow a healthy diet, as weight gain can occur with long-term use. › Monitor for manifestations of increased depression and intent of suicide.
Sedative Hypnotic Anxiolytics (Benzodiazepines)	
› Diazepam (Valium) › Lorazepam (Ativan)	› Observe for CNS depression, such as sedation, lightheadedness, ataxia, and decreased cognitive function. › Avoid the use of other CNS depressants, such as alcohol. › Avoid hazardous activities (driving, operating heavy equipment/machinery). › Caffeine interferes with the desired effects of the medication. › Advise the client who wants to discontinue a benzodiazepine to seek the advice of a provider. These medications should not be abruptly discontinued. The dosage should be gradually tapered over several weeks.
Mood stabilizers	
› Lithium carbonate (Lithobid)	› Gastrointestinal effects may be minimized by taking medication with food or milk. › Maintain a healthy diet, and exercise regularly to minimize weight gain. › Maintain fluid intake of 2 to 3 L/day from food and beverage sources. › Maintain adequate sodium intake. › Encourage the client to comply with laboratory appointments needed to monitor lithium effectiveness and adverse effects.
Antiepileptics	
› Valproic acid (Depakote)	› Take medication with food to minimize gastrointestinal discomfort.
Atypical antipsychotics	
› Risperidone (Risperdal) › Olanzapine (Zyprexa)	› To minimize weight gain, advise the client to maintain a healthy diet and exercise regularly. › Instruct the client to report clinical findings of agitation, dizziness, sedation, and sleep disruption to the provider, as the medication may need to be changed.

- Care After Discharge
  - Nursing Actions
    - Ask the client to agree to a no-suicide contract, which is a verbal or written agreement that the client makes to not harm himself, but instead to seek help.
      - A no-suicide contract is not legally binding and should only be used according to facility policy.
      - A no-suicide contract may be beneficial, but it should not replace other suicide prevention strategies.
      - A no-suicide contract can be used as a tool to develop and maintain trust between the nurse and the client.
      - A no-suicide contract is discouraged for clients who are in crisis, under the influence of substances, psychotic, very impulsive, or very angry/agitated. A contract does not take the place of suicide precautions.
- Client Education
  - Assist the client to develop a support-system list with specific names, agencies, and telephone numbers that the client can call in case of an emergency.

APPLICATION EXERCISES

1. A nurse is collecting data from a client at a community mental health facility using the SAD PERSONS tool. The nurse knows that this tool provides which of the following data related to a client?

    A. Current anxiety level

    B. Problem-solving ability

    C. Suicide potential

    D. Mood disturbance

2. A client says, "I plan to commit suicide." Which of the following should be the nurse's priority when collecting data?

    A. Client's educational and economic background

    B. Lethality of the method and availability of means

    C. Quality of the client's social support

    D. Client's insight into the reasons for the decision

3. A nurse is collecting data from a client who is suicidal. Which of the following are appropriate for the nurse to ask the client? (Select all that apply.)

    _____ A. "Do you have a plan?"

    _____ B. "Have you thought about hurting yourself?"

    _____ C. "Do you feel that life is not worth living?"

    _____ D. "Why do you want to commit suicide?"

    _____ E. "Have you experienced a recent change in your mood?"

4. A nurse is assisting with the plan of care for a client who is on suicide precautions. Which of the following interventions should the nurse include in the plan of care?

    A. Assign the client to a private room.

    B. Document the client's behavior every hour.

    C. Allow the client to keep perfume in her room.

    D. Ensure that the client swallows medication.

5. A nurse is caring for a client who has a new prescription for sertraline (Zoloft). Use the ATI Active Learning Template: Medication and the ATI Pharmacology Review Module to complete this item to include:

    A. Side/Adverse Effects: Identify four.

    B. Nursing Interventions/Client Education: Describe at least three nursing interventions/client education.

APPLICATION EXERCISES KEY

1. A. INCORRECT: SAD PERSONS does not provide data related to the client's current anxiety level.

    B. INCORRECT: SAD PERSONS does not provide data related to a client's ability to problem solve.

    C. **CORRECT:** SAD PERSONS provides data related to a client's suicide potential.

    D. INCORRECT: SAD PERSONS does not provide data related to a client's mood disturbance.

    Ⓝ NCLEX® Connection: Psychosocial Integrity, Crisis Intervention

2. A. INCORRECT: This is an appropriate action by the nurse. However, it is not the priority.

    B. **CORRECT:** The greatest risk to the client is self-harm as a result of carrying out a suicide plan. Therefore, the priority when collecting data is to determine how lethal the method is, how available the method is, and how detailed the plan is.

    C. INCORRECT: This is an appropriate action by the nurse. However, it is not the priority.

    D. INCORRECT: This is an appropriate action by the nurse. However, it is not the priority.

    Ⓝ NCLEX® Connection: Psychosocial Integrity, Crisis Intervention

3. A. **CORRECT:** It is important to ask the client if she has a plan.

    B. **CORRECT:** The nurse should ask the client about thoughts of hurting herself.

    C. **CORRECT:** This is an appropriate question for nurse to ask a client who is suicidal.

    D. INCORRECT: This is a nontherapeutic response. "Why" questions should be avoided because they may cause the client to be defensive.

    E. **CORRECT:** This is an appropriate question for the nurse to ask a client who is suicidal.

    Ⓝ NCLEX® Connection: Psychosocial Integrity, Crisis Intervention

4. A. INCORRECT: Clients who are suicidal should not be assigned a private room.

    B. INCORRECT: The client's behavior should be documented every 15 minutes.

    C. INCORRECT: Remove perfume from the client's room.

    D. **CORRECT:** Ensure that the client swallows medication.

    Ⓝ NCLEX® Connection: Psychosocial Integrity, Crisis Intervention

5. *Using the ATI Active Learning Template: Medication*

    A. Side/Adverse Effects
    - Nausea
    - Headache
    - CNS stimulation (agitation, insomnia, anxiety)
    - Sexual dysfunction

    B. Nursing Interventions/Client Education
    - Do not stop taking medication suddenly.
    - Medications can take 1 to 3 weeks for therapeutic effects for initial response, with up to 2 months for maximal response.
    - Avoid hazardous activities (driving, operating heavy equipment/machinery) until medication side effects are known.
    - Follow a healthy diet, as weight gain can occur with long-term use.
    - Monitor for clinical findings of increased depression and intent of suicide.

    Ⓝ NCLEX® Connection: Pharmacological Therapies, Adverse Effects/Contraindications/ Side Effects/Interactions

chapter 29

Overview

- Anger, a normal feeling, is an emotional response to frustration as perceived by the individual. It can be positive if there is truly an unfair or wrong situation that needs to be righted.

- Anger becomes negative when it is denied, suppressed, or expressed inappropriately, such as by using aggressive behavior.

  ○ Denied or suppressed anger can manifest as physical or psychological findings, such as headaches, coronary artery disease, hypertension, gastric ulcers, depression, or low self-esteem.

- Aggression, unlike anger, is typically goal-directed with the intent of harming a specific person or object.

  ○ Inappropriately expressed anger can become hostility or aggression.

  ○ Aggression includes physical or verbal responses that indicate rage and potential harm to self, others, or property.

  ○ A client who is often angry and aggressive can have underlying feelings of inadequacy, insecurity, guilt, fear, and rejection.

- Comorbidities include depressive disorders, posttraumatic stress disorder (PTSD), Alzheimer's disease, and personality and psychotic disorders.

- Categories/Taxonomies of Disorder

  ○ Preassaultive – The client begins to become angry and exhibits increasing anxiety, hyperactivity, and verbal abuse.

  ○ Assaultive – The client commits an act of violence. Seclusion and physical restraints can be required.

  ○ Postassaultive – Staff reviews the incident with the client during this stage.

- Despite the potential for anger and aggression among individuals who have mental illness, it is important to know that individuals who have a mental illness are more likely to hurt themselves than to express aggression against others.

- Seclusion and restraint must be used only according to legal guidelines and should be the interventions of last resort after other less restrictive options have been tried.

- New initiatives are being proposed to reduce or eliminate the use of mechanical restraints. National, state, and local initiatives advocate for restraint elimination. There is also heightened awareness of the damaging effects restraints may have on clients, clinicians, and caretakers alike.

  ○ Seclusion and restraint do not usually lead to positive behavior change. Seclusion and restraint may keep individuals safe during a violent outburst, but the use of restraint itself can be dangerous and has, on rare occasions, led to the death of clients due to reasons such as suffocation and strangulation.

  ○ Intramuscular medication can need to be given if aggression is threatening and if no medications were previously given.

  ○ When deemed essential to use restraints, remove the client from seclusion or restraint as soon as the crisis is over and when the client attempts reconciliation and is no longer aggressive.

Data Collection

- Risk Factors
  - Past history of aggression, poor impulse control, and violence
  - Poor coping skills, limited support systems
  - Comorbidity that leads to acts of violence (psychotic delusions, command hallucinations, violent angry reactions with cognitive disorders)
  - Living in a violent environment
  - Inadequate limit setting by the nurse within the therapeutic milieu
- Subjective and Objective Data
  - Hyperactivity such as pacing, restlessness
  - Defensive response when criticized, easily offended
  - Eye contact that is intense, or no eye contact at all
  - Facial expressions, such as frowning or grimacing
  - Body language, such as clenching fists, waving arms
  - Rapid breathing
  - Aggressive postures, such as leaning forward, appearing tense
  - Verbal clues, such as loud, rapid talking
  - Drug or alcohol intoxication

Patient-Centered Care

- Nursing Care
  - Provide a safe environment for the client who is aggressive, as well as for the other clients and staff on the unit.
  - Follow policies of the mental health setting when working with clients who demonstrate aggression.
  - Identify triggers or preconditions that escalate client emotion.
  - Steps to handle aggressive and/or escalating behavior in a mental health setting include the following.
    - Responding quickly
    - Remaining calm and in control
    - Encouraging the client to express feelings verbally, using therapeutic communication techniques (reflective techniques, silence, active listening)
      - Communicating with honesty and sincerity
      - Avoiding accusatory or threatening statements
    - Allowing the client as much personal space as possible
    - Maintaining eye contact and sitting or standing at the same level as the client with a nonaggressive stance
    - Describing options clearly and offering the client choices
    - Reassuring the client that staff are present to help prevent loss of control

- Setting limits for the client
  - ◻ Tell the client calmly and directly what he must do in a particular situation, such as, "I need you to stop yelling and walk with me to the day room where we can talk."
  - ◻ Use physical activity, such as walking, to de-escalate anger and behaviors.
  - ◻ Inform the client of the consequences of his behavior, such as loss of privileges.
- Use pharmacological interventions if the client does not respond to calm limit setting.
- Plan for four to six staff members to be available and in sight of the client as a "show of force" if appropriate.
- ○ Following an aggressive/violent episode
  - Discuss ways for the client to keep control during the aggression cycle.
  - Encourage the client to talk about the incident, and what triggered and escalated the aggression from the client's perspective.
  - Participate in staff debriefing to evaluate the effectiveness of actions.
  - Document the entire incident completely by including:
    - ◻ Behaviors leading up to, as well as those observed throughout the critical incident.
    - ◻ Nursing interventions implemented, and the client's response.
- Medications
  - ○ Olanzapine (Zyprexa)
  - ○ Ziprasidone (Geodon)
    - Classification and therapeutic intent
      - ◻ Olanzapine and ziprasidone are atypical antipsychotics used to control aggressive and impulsive behaviors. These are used more commonly than haloperidol because of the severity of adverse effects of haloperidol.
  - ○ Haloperidol (Haldol)
    - Classification and therapeutic intent
      - ◻ Haloperidol is an antipsychotic agent used to control aggressive and impulsive behavior.
    - Nursing considerations
      - ◻ Monitor for clinical findings of parkinsonism and anticholinergic adverse effects.
      - ◻ Keep client hydrated, check vital signs, and test for muscle rigidity due to the risk of neuroleptic malignant syndrome (NMS).

  - ○ Other medications may be used to prevent violent behavior by treating the underlying disorder. These include antidepressants, such as SSRIs; mood stabilizers, such as lithium; and sedative/hypnotic medications, such as benzodiazepines.
- Care After Discharge and Client Education
  - ○ Nursing Actions
    - Reinforce teaching about medications.
    - Assist the client to develop problem-solving skills.
    - Encourage the client to return for follow up.
    - Encourage the client to attend a support group.

APPLICATION EXERCISES

1. A nurse is assisting with group therapy for a group of clients. Which of the following statements made by a client is an example of aggressive communication?

    A. "I wish you would not make me angry."

    B. "I feel angry when you leave me."

    C. "It makes me angry when you interrupt me."

    D. "You'd better listen to me."

2. A nurse is caring for a client who is speaking in a loud voice with clenched fists. Which of the following actions should the nurse take?

    A. Demand that the client stop yelling.

    B. Request that other staff members remain close by.

    C. Move as close to the client as possible.

    D. Walk away from the client.

3. A nurse is collecting data on a client in an acute mental health unit. Which of the following findings should the nurse expect if the client is in the preassaultive stage of violence? (Select all that apply.)

    _____ A. Lethargy

    _____ B. Defensive responses to questions

    _____ C. Disorientation

    _____ D. Rapid breathing

    _____ E. Facial grimacing

    _____ F. Agitation

4. A nurse is caring for a client in an acute mental health facility who gets up from a chair and throws it across the day room. Which of the following is the priority nursing action?

    A. Encourage the client to express her feelings.

    B. Maintain eye contact with the client.

    C. Move the client away from others.

    D. Tell the client that the behavior is not acceptable.

5. A nurse is caring for a client who is screaming at staff members and other clients. Which of the following is a therapeutic response by the nurse to this client?

    A. "Stop screaming, and walk with me outside."

    B. "Why are you so angry and screaming at everyone?"

    C. "You will not get your way by screaming."

    D. "You do know that screaming is unacceptable behavior?"

6. A nurse is caring for a client who hit another client. The nurse is preparing to administer haloperidol (Haldol). Use the ATI Active Learning Template: Medication and the ATI Pharmacology Review Module to complete this item to include the following sections:

    A. Expected Pharmacological Action

    B. Side/Adverse Effects: Identify at least four.

    C. Nursing Interventions/Client Education: Describe at least four.

APPLICATION EXERCISES KEY

1. A. INCORRECT: This statement does not imply a threat, nor does it indicate a lack of respect for another individual.

    B. INCORRECT: This statement does not imply a threat, nor does it indicate a lack of respect for another individual.

    C. INCORRECT: This statement does not imply a threat, nor does it indicate a lack of respect for another individual.

    D. **CORRECT:** This statement implies a threat and a lack of respect for another individual.

    (N) NCLEX® Connection: Psychosocial Integrity, Behavioral Management

2. A. INCORRECT: The nurse should not make demands of the client. This nontherapeutic approach could increase the client's aggression.

    B. **CORRECT:** The nurse should request that other staff members remain close by to assist if necessary.

    C. INCORRECT: Angry clients need a large personal space.

    D. INCORRECT: The nurse should never walk away from an angry client. It is the nurse's responsibility to intervene as appropriate.

    (N) NCLEX® Connection: Psychosocial Integrity, Crisis Intervention

3. A. INCORRECT: Lethargy is an expected finding of a client who has depression.

    B. **CORRECT:** Defensive responses to questions can indicate that a client is in the preassaultive stage of violence.

    C. INCORRECT: Disorientation is an expected finding of a client who has a cognitive disorder.

    D. **CORRECT:** Rapid breathing can indicate that a client is in the preassaultive stage of violence.

    E. **CORRECT:** Facial grimacing can indicate that a client is in the preassaultive stage of violence.

    F. **CORRECT:** Agitation can indicate that a client is in the preassaultive stage of violence.

    (N) NCLEX® Connection: Psychosocial Integrity, Crisis Intervention

4. A. INCORRECT: Encouraging the client to express her feelings is appropriate. However, it is not the priority action.

    B. INCORRECT: Maintaining eye contact with the client is appropriate. However, it is not the priority action.

    C. **CORRECT:** The client's actions indicate the greatest risk is injury to others. Therefore, the priority action is to move the client away from others.

    D. INCORRECT: Telling the client that the behavior is not acceptable is appropriate. However, it is not the priority action.

    Ⓝ NCLEX® Connection: Safety and Infection Control, Accident/Error/Injury Prevention

5. A. **CORRECT:** This is an appropriate therapeutic response. Setting limits and the use of physical activity, such as walking, to de-escalate anger is an appropriate intervention.

    B. INCORRECT: "Why" questions imply criticism and will often cause the client to become defensive.

    C. INCORRECT: This is a closed-ended, nontherapeutic statement.

    D. INCORRECT: This is a closed-ended, nontherapeutic statement.

    Ⓝ NCLEX® Connection: Psychosocial Integrity, Behavioral Management

6. *Using the ATI Active Learning Template: Medication*

    A. Expected Pharmacological Action
    - Haloperidol is an antipsychotic agent used to control aggressive and impulsive behavior.

    B. Side/Adverse Effects
    - Sedation
    - Orthostatic hypotension
    - Extrapyramidal symptoms (EPS)
      - Acute dystonia
      - Parkinsonism
      - Akathisia
      - Tardive dyskinesia
    - Anticholinergic adverse effects
      - Dry mouth
      - Blurred vision
      - Constipation
      - Photophobia
      - Urinary hesitancy or retention

    C. Nursing Interventions/Client Education
    - Encourage the client to drink frequent sips of water and chew gum.
    - Instruct the client to increase fiber intake and that a stool softener may be needed.
    - Instruct the client to limit sunlight exposure, and encourage wearing sunscreen and sunglasses.
    - Advise the client to void just before taking medication.
    - Monitor the client for indications of EPS
    - Monitor blood pressure and heart rate.
    - Protect the client from injury or falls.

    Ⓝ NCLEX® Connection: Pharmacological Therapies, Expected Actions/Outcomes

chapter 30

Overview

- Violence from one person toward another is a social act involving a serious abuse of power. Usually, a relatively stronger person controls or injures another, typically the least powerful person accessible to the abuser. This includes acts of violence that a spouse commits against another spouse, a parent against a child, or a child against a parent.
  - A nurse must prepare to deal with various types of violence and the mental health consequences.
    - Violence can be directed toward a family member, a stranger, or an acquaintance. Or, it can come from a human-made mass-casualty incident, such as a terrorist attack.
    - Natural disasters, such as hurricanes and earthquakes, can cause mental health effects comparable to those caused by human-made violence.
    - Violence against a person who has a mental illness is more likely to occur when factors such as poverty, transient lifestyle, or a substance use disorder are present.
    - A person who has a mental illness is no more likely to harm strangers than anyone else.
    - The factor most likely to predict violence between strangers is a past history of violence and criminal activity.

Data Collection

- Risk Factors
  - A female partner is the victim in the majority of family violence, but the male partner also can be a victim of violence.
  - Victims are at the greatest risk for violence when they try to leave the relationship.
  - Pregnancy tends to increase the likelihood of violence toward the intimate partner. The reason for this is unclear.
  - Factors that increase the risk for abuse toward a child
    - The child is under 3 years of age
    - A perpetrator perceives the child as being different (the child is the result of an unwanted pregnancy, is physically disabled, or has some other trait that makes him particularly vulnerable)

  - Older or other adults who are vulnerable within the home can suffer abuse because they are in poor health, exhibit disruptive behavior, or are dependent on a caregiver. The potential for violence against an older adult is highest in families where violence has already occurred.

- Violence is most common within family groups, and most is aimed at family and friends rather than strangers.
  - Family violence occurs across all economic and educational backgrounds and racial and ethnic groups in the United States. It is often termed "maltreatment."
  - Family violence or maltreatment can occur against children, intimate partners, or vulnerable adult family members.
  - Within the family, a cycle of violence can occur between intimate (domestic) partners.
    - Tension-building phase – The abuser has minor episodes of anger and can be verbally abusive and responsible for some minor physical violence. The victim is tense during this stage and tends to accept the blame for what is happening.
    - Acute battering phase – The tension becomes too much to bear and serious abuse takes place. The victim can try to cover up the injury or can get help.
    - Honeymoon phase – The situation is defused for awhile after the violent episode. The abuser becomes loving, promises to change, and is sorry for the behavior. The victim wants to believe this and hopes for a change. Eventually, the cycle begins again.
    - Periods of escalation and de-escalation usually continue, with shorter and shorter periods of time between the two. Emotions for the abuser and victim, such as fear or anger, increase in intensity. Repeated episodes of violence lead to feelings of powerlessness.

  - Cultural differences can influence whether or not the nursing data is valid, how the client responds to interventions, and the appropriateness of nursing interactions with the client.
- Types of Violence
  - Physical violence occurs when physical pain or harm is directed:
    - Toward an infant or child, as is the case with shaken baby syndrome (caused by violent shaking of young infants).
    - Toward an intimate partner, such as striking or strangling the partner.
    - Toward a vulnerable adult in the home, such as pushing an older adult parent and causing her to fall.
  - Sexual violence occurs when sexual contact takes place without consent, whether the victim is able or unable to give that consent.
  - Emotional violence includes behavior that minimizes an individual's feelings of self-worth or humiliates, threatens, or intimidates a family member.
  - Neglect, which includes the failure to provide the following.
    - Physical care, such as feeding
    - Emotional care, such as interacting with a child, or stimulation necessary for a child to develop normally
    - An education for a child, such as enrolling a young child in school
    - Necessary health or dental care
  - Economic maltreatment
    - Failure to provide for the needs of a victim when adequate funds are available
    - Unpaid bills, resulting in disconnection of heat or electricity

- Vulnerable person (victim) characteristics
  - Demonstration of low self-esteem and feelings of helplessness, hopelessness, powerlessness, guilt, and shame
  - Attempts to protect the perpetrator and accept responsibility for the abuse
  - Possible denial of the severity of the situation and feelings of anger and terror
- Perpetrator characteristics
  - Possible use of threats and intimidation to control the victim
  - Is usually an extreme disciplinarian who believes in physical punishment
  - Possible history of substance use disorder
  - Has difficulty assuming typical adult roles
  - Is likely to have experienced family violence as a child
- Age-Specific Assessments
  - Infants
    - Shaken baby syndrome – Shaking can cause intracranial hemorrhage. Monitor for respiratory distress, bulging fontanelles, and an increase in head circumference. Retinal hemorrhage can be present.
    - Any bruising on an infant before age 6 months is suspicious.
  - Preschoolers to adolescents
    - Check for unusual bruising, such as on abdomen, back, or buttocks. Bruising is common on arms and legs in these age groups.
    - Check the mechanism of injury, which might not be congruent with the physical appearance of the injury. Numerous bruises at different stages of healing can indicate ongoing beatings. Be suspicious of bruises or welts that resemble the shape of a belt buckle or other object.
    - Check for burns. Burns covering "glove" or "stocking" areas of the hands or feet can indicate forced immersion into boiling water. Small, round burns can be from lit cigarettes.
    - Check for fractures with unusual features, such as forearm spiral fractures, which could be a result of twisting the extremity forcefully. The presence of multiple fractures is suspicious.
    - Check for human bite marks.
    - Check for head injuries – level of consciousness, equal and reactive pupils, and nausea or vomiting.

  - Older and other vulnerable adults
    - Monitor for any bruises, lacerations, abrasions, or fractures in which the physical appearance does not match the history or mechanism of injury.

Patient-Centered Care

- Nursing Care
  - All states have mandatory reporting laws that require nurses to report suspected abuse. There are civil and criminal penalties for not reporting suspicions of abuse.
  - Nursing interventions for child or vulnerable adult abuse must include the following.
    - Mandatory reporting of suspected or actual cases of child or vulnerable adult abuse.
    - Complete and accurate documentation of subjective and objective data obtained during data collection.

- A forensic nurse has advanced training in the collection of evidence for suspected or actual cases of sexual assault or other forms of physical abuse.
- Assist with conducting a nursing history.
  - Provide privacy when conducting interviews about family abuse.
  - Be direct, honest, and professional.
  - Use language the client understands.
  - Be understanding and attentive.
  - Use therapeutic techniques that demonstrate understanding.
  - Use open-ended questions to elicit descriptive responses.
  - Inform the client if a referral must be made to child or adult protective services, and be sure to explain the process.
- Provide basic care to treat injuries.
- Make appropriate referrals.
- Nursing interventions for community-wide or mass casualty incidents, such as a school shooting or gang violence.
  - Early intervention
    - Provide psychological first aid.
      - Make sure clients are physically and psychologically safe from harm.
      - Reduce stress-related symptoms, such as using techniques to alleviate a panic attack.
      - Provide interventions to restore rest and sleep, and provide links to social supports and information about critical resources.
    - Depending on their level of expertise and training, mental health nurses can collect data; provide consultation; and provide therapeutic communication and support, triage, and psychological and physical care.
  - Critical incident stress debriefing

    - This is a crisis intervention strategy that assists clients who have experienced a traumatic event, usually involving violence (staff experiencing client violence, school children and personnel experiencing the violent death of a student, rescue workers after an earthquake) in a safe environment.
    - Debriefing can take place in group meetings with a facilitator who promotes a safe environment where there can be expression of thoughts and feelings.
    - The facilitator will acknowledge reactions, provide anticipatory guidance for symptoms that can still occur, teach stress management techniques, and provide referrals.
    - The group can choose to meet on an ongoing basis or disband after resolution of the crisis.
- Trauma-specific interventions

  - Trauma Affect Regulation: Guide for Education and Therapy (TARGET) – Provides trauma survivors with a therapeutic approach to healing while offering education about practical skills to manage emotions and the effect of memories on daily life.
  - Trauma Recovery and Empowerment Model (TREM) – A gender-specific model (TREM for female and M-TREM for male) designed to assist survivors of trauma, specifically physical or sexual trauma.

- Care After Discharge

  - Nursing Actions
    - Help client develop a safety plan, identify behaviors and situations that might trigger violence, and provide information regarding safe places to live.
    - Encourage participation in support groups.
    - Use case management to coordinate community, medical, criminal justice, and social services.
    - Use crisis intervention techniques to help resolve family or community situations where violence has been devastating.
  - Client Education
    - Instruct clients regarding normal growth and development.
    - Inform clients of self-care and empowerment skills.
    - Discuss with clients ways to manage stress.

APPLICATION EXERCISES

1. A nurse is assisting with leading a peer group discussion about family and community violence. Which of the following statements by a member of the group indicates a need for further teaching?

    A. "A criminal history increases the risk for violence between strangers."

    B. "Substance use disorder increases the risk for violence."

    C. "Entering an intimate relationship increases the risk for violence."

    D. "Pregnancy increases the risk for violence toward the intimate partner."

2. A nurse is caring for an adult client who is the victim of intimate partner abuse. The client does not wish to report the violence to law enforcement authorities. Which of the following nursing actions is the highest priority?

    A. Advise the client about the location of women's shelters.

    B. Encourage the client to participate in a support group for victims of abuse.

    C. Implement case management to coordinate community and social services.

    D. Tell the client about the use of stress management techniques.

3. A nurse is preparing to collect data on an infant who has shaken baby syndrome. Which of the following is an expected finding? (Select all that apply.)

    _____ A. Sunken fontanelles

    _____ B. Respiratory distress

    _____ C. Retinal hemorrhage

    _____ D. Altered level of consciousness

    _____ E. An increase in head circumference

4. A nurse working in an emergency department is checking a child who reports abdominal pain. When collecting data, which of the following findings should alert the nurse to possible abuse? (Select all that apply.)

    _____ A. Abrasions on knees

    _____ B. Round burn marks on forearms

    _____ C. Mismatched clothing

    _____ D. Abdominal rebound tenderness

    _____ E. Areas of ecchymosis on torso

5. A nurse is preparing a community education seminar about family violence. When discussing the types of violence, the nurse should include which of the following?

    A. Refusing to pay bills for a dependant, even when funds are available, is neglect.

    B. Intentionally causing an older adult to fall is an example of physical violence.

    C. Striking an intimate partner is an example of sexual violence.

    D. Failure to provide a stimulating environment for normal development is emotional abuse.

6. A nurse is discussing intimate partner abuse with a newly licensed nurse. Use the ATI Active Learning Template: Basic Concept to complete this item to include the following sections:

    A. Underlying Principles:
- Discuss the three phases in the cycle of violence.
- Identify at least three characteristics of a vulnerable person (victim).
- Identify at least three characteristics of a perpetrator.

    B. Nursing Interventions:
- Identify at least four appropriate nursing actions when conducting a nursing history.

APPLICATION EXERCISES KEY

1. A. INCORRECT: This statement does not require further teaching. A past history of violence or criminal activity is a common risk factor for violence between strangers.

    B. INCORRECT: This statement does not require further teaching. Substance use disorder increases the risk for violence.

    C. **CORRECT:** This statement requires further teaching. Victims are at the greatest risk for violence when they try to leave the relationship.

    D. INCORRECT: This statement does not require further teaching. Pregnancy tends to increase the likelihood of violence toward the intimate partner.

    (N) NCLEX® Connection: Psychosocial Integrity, Abuse/Neglect

2. A. **CORRECT:** The client's safety is the highest priority. Therefore, the development of a safety plan that includes the identification of safe places to live is the priority nursing action.

    B. INCORRECT: It is appropriate to encourage participation in a support group. However, this does not address the greatest risk to the client and is therefore not the priority nursing action.

    C. INCORRECT: It is appropriate to implement case management. However, this does not address the greatest risk to the client and is therefore not the priority nursing action.

    D. INCORRECT: It is appropriate to tell the client about the use of stress management techniques. However, this does not address the greatest risk to the client and is therefore not the priority nursing action.

    (N) NCLEX® Connection: Psychosocial Integrity, Abuse/Neglect

3. A. INCORRECT: Bulging, rather than sunken, fontanelles are an expected finding of shaken baby syndrome.

    B. **CORRECT:** Respiratory distress is an expected finding of shaken baby syndrome.

    C. **CORRECT:** Retinal hemorrhage is an expected finding of shaken baby syndrome.

    D. **CORRECT:** An altered level of consciousness is an expected finding of shaken baby syndrome due to intracranial trauma or hemorrhage.

    E. **CORRECT:** An increase in head circumference is an expected finding of shaken baby syndrome.

    (N) NCLEX® Connection: Psychosocial Integrity, Abuse/Neglect

4. A. INCORRECT: Minor injuries on the arms and legs, such as abrasions, are common in this age group.

   B. **CORRECT:** Round burn marks anywhere on the child's body can indicate cigarette burns and should alert the nurse to possible abuse.

   C. INCORRECT: Mismatched clothing is consistent with the child's developmental age.

   D. INCORRECT: Abdominal rebound tenderness is a possible indication of appendicitis rather than abuse.

   E. **CORRECT:** Areas of ecchymosis on the torso, back, or buttocks should alert the nurse to possible abuse.

   (N) NCLEX® Connection: Psychosocial Integrity, Abuse/Neglect

5. A. INCORRECT: Refusing to pay bills for a dependant is economic maltreatment, rather than neglect.

   B. **CORRECT:** Physical violence occurs when physical pain or harm is directed toward another individual.

   C. INCORRECT: Striking an intimate partner or other individual is an example of physical, rather than sexual, violence. Sexual violence occurs when sexual contact takes place without consent.

   D. INCORRECT: Failure to provide a stimulating environment for normal development is neglect, rather than emotional abuse.

   (N) NCLEX® Connection: Psychosocial Integrity, Abuse/Neglect

6. *Using the ATI Active Learning Template: Basic Concept*

   A. Underlying Principles
   - Cycle of violence
     - Tension-building phase – The initial phase when the perpetrator has minor episodes of anger and can inflict verbal abuse or minor physical violence. The victim is tense and can accept the blame for what is happening.
     - Acute battering phase – The tension reaches a peak and a serious battering incident occurs. The victim can try to cover up the injury or seek help.
     - Honeymoon phase – The abuser is sorry for the behavior and promises to change. The victim wants to believe the abuser and hopes for a change.
   - Characteristics of a vulnerable person
     - Feelings of low self-esteem, helplessness, hopelessness, powerlessness, guilt, and shame
     - Attempts to protect the perpetrator and accept responsibility for the abuse
     - Possible denial of the severity of the situation
     - Feelings of anger and terror
   - Characteristics of a perpetrator
     - Uses threats and intimidation to control the vulnerable individual
     - Extreme disciplinarian who uses physical punishment
     - Possible history of substance use disorder
     - Possible history of family violence as a child
     - Difficulty assuming adult roles

   B. Nursing Interventions
   - Provide a safe and private environment to conduct the interview.
   - Be direct, honest, and professional.
   - Use language that the client understands.
   - Be understanding and attentive.
   - Use therapeutic communication.

   (N) NCLEX® Connection: Psychosocial Integrity, Abuse/Neglect

REFERENCES

Dudek, S. G. (2010). *Nutrition essentials for nursing practice* (6th ed.). Philadelphia: Lippincott Williams & Wilkins.

Ford, S. M., & Roach, S. S. (2013). *Roach's introductory clinical pharmacology* (10th ed.). Philadelphia: Lippincott Williams & Wilkins.

Grodner, M., Roth, S. L., & Walkingshaw, B. C. (2012). *Nutrition foundations and clinical applications of nutrition: A nursing approach* (5th ed.). St. Louis, MO: Mosby.

Hockenberry, M. J., & Winkelstein M. L. (2013). *Wong's essentials of pediatric nursing* (9th ed.). St. Louis, MO: Mosby.

Lehne, R. A. (2013). *Pharmacology for nursing care* (8th ed.). St. Louis: Saunders.

Townsend, M. C. (2011). *Essentials of psychiatric mental health nursing: Concepts of care in evidence-based practice* (5th ed.). Philadelphia: F. A. Davis.

Varcarolis, E. M., Carson, V. B., & Shoemaker, N. C. (2010). *Foundations of psychiatric mental health nursing: A clinical approach* (6th ed.). St. Louis, MO: Saunders.

Wilson, B. A., Shannon, M. T., & Shields, K. M. (2013). *Pearson nurse's drug guide 2013*. Upper Saddle River, NJ: Prentice Hall.

Appendix

CONTENT_____ REVIEW MODULE CHAPTER _____

TOPIC DESCRIPTOR_____

Related Content	Underlying Principles	Nursing Interventions
(e.g. delegation, levels of prevention, advance directives)		› Who? › When? › Why? › How?

Appendix

CONTENT_____ REVIEW MODULE CHAPTER _____

TOPIC DESCRIPTOR_____

DESCRIPTION OF PROCEDURE:

Procedure Name

Indications

Interpretation of Findings

Nursing Interventions (pre, intra, post)

Potential Complications

Nursing Interventions

Client Education

Appendix

CONTENT _____ REVIEW MODULE CHAPTER _____

TOPIC DESCRIPTOR _____

Alteration in Health (Diagnosis)	Client Problem Related to Alteration in Health	Pathophysiology Related to Client Problem

Safety Considerations

Assessment

- Past Medical History
- Medications
- Risk Factors
- Laboratory Data
- Objective and Subjective Data
- Diagnostic Procedures/ Surgical Interventions

Teamwork and Collaboration

- Discharge Planning
- Interprofessional Care
- Coordination of Client Care

Nursing Interventions (Evidence-Based)

Client Education

Outcomes/Evaluations

Appendix

CONTENT_____ REVIEW MODULE CHAPTER _____

TOPIC DESCRIPTOR_____

```
                        ┌────────────────────────────────┐
                        │      Developmental Stage        │
                        └────────────────────────────────┘
```

Physical Development	Cognitive Development	Age-Appropriate Activities

```
                        ┌────────────────────────────────┐
                        │       Health Promotion          │
                        └────────────────────────────────┘
```

Immunizations	Health Screening	Nutrition	Injury Prevention

APPENDIX   ACTIVE LEARNING TEMPLATES

TEMPLATE   Medication

CONTENT _____ REVIEW MODULE CHAPTER _____

TOPIC DESCRIPTOR_____

MEDICATION _____

EXPECTED PHARMALOGICAL ACTION:

```
┌──────────────────────────────────────────┐
│             Therapeutic Uses              │
│                                           │
└──────────────────────────────────────────┘

┌───────────────────────┐   ┌───────────────────────┐
│    Adverse Effects     │   │  Nursing Interventions │
│                        │   │                        │
│                        │   │                        │
└───────────────────────┘   │                        │
┌───────────────────────┐   └───────────────────────┘
│    Contraindications    │
│                        │   ┌───────────────────────┐
│                        │   │   Client Education     │
└───────────────────────┘   │                        │
┌───────────────────────┐   │                        │
│ Medication/Food        │   │                        │
│ Interactions           │   └───────────────────────┘
│                        │
└───────────────────────┘

┌───────────────────────┐   ┌───────────────────────┐
│ Medication             │   │ Evaluation of          │
│ Administration         │   │ Medication             │
│                        │   │ Effectiveness          │
└───────────────────────┘   └───────────────────────┘
```

Appendix

CONTENT_____ REVIEW MODULE CHAPTER_____

TOPIC DESCRIPTOR_____

DESCRIPTION OF SKILL:

Procedure Name

Indications

Nursing Interventions
(pre, intra, post)

Outcomes/Evaluations

Potential Complications

Nursing Interventions

Client Education

Appendix

CONTENT _____ REVIEW MODULE CHAPTER _____

TOPIC DESCRIPTOR_____

DESCRIPTION OF PROCEDURE:

Procedure Name

Indications

Nursing Interventions
(pre, intra, post)

Outcomes/Evaluations

Potential Complications

Nursing Interventions

Client Education